What People Are Saying

"*A Size That Fits* is a thoughtful, informative and well-crafted book that will help readers break through the noise, frustration, and failure of past weight loss attempts and lifestyle changes. Throughout the book Dr. Creel eloquently reminds us how to find hidden success and lessons with every failure. By emphasizing the value of mindfulness and self-awareness on the journey toward a more positive long-term lifestyle, he challenges readers to look beyond numbers on the scales and the tags on their clothing. Although written for patients, Dr. Creel's book is an excellent resource for healthcare professionals who seek a real-life approach to support their clients."

–*Kellene A. Isom, MS, RD, LDN, CAGS (Bariatric Program Director, Center for Metabolic Health and Bariatric Surgery Brigham and Women's Hospital / Brigham and Women's Faulkner Hospital, and CDR Representative at the Commission on Dietetic Registration)*

"In *A Size That Fits*, David Creel presents a realistic and holistic strategy to help you reach weight loss and fitness goals. This is not a rigid, restrictive, quick-fix one-size-fits-all diet plan where lost pounds quickly return. Instead, he explores how thoughts, emotion, genetics, hormones, environment, stress, unrealistic expectations, accomplishments, failure, and habits helped *shape* the shape you're in. He then equips you with practical, evidence-based tools and strategies to lose weight, look better, feel better, and live better."

–*Patrick Perry, MPH, Executive Editor*, The Saturday Evening Post *magazine*

"This is the first weight management book that has ever worked for me. Thank you, Dr. Creel!"

–*Sammie Justesen, RN, publisher, NorLights Press*

D1509133

NorLightsPress
762 State Road 458
Bedford, IN 47421

Printed in the United States of America
ISBN: 978-0-9976834-6-2

Book Design and Editing: Sammie and Vorris Dee Justesen
Interior by Praditha Kahatapitiya
Cover Design: Colton Creel and Kiryl Lysenka

First printing, 2017

Note: In order to respect the privacy of past clients, the author has altered names and some descriptive details. At times he has combined several patients' experiences into one event. Unless described as such, none of the experiences in this book are purely fictional. This book is intended for educational purposes and is not a substitute for medical or psychiatric treatment. Please consult with a qualified medical professional before attempting weight loss.

Dedication

This book is dedicated to my parents, who taught me to live with deep character. Although I didn't always listen or follow in your footsteps, thank you for showing me the way.

About the Book Cover and Title

THE BOOK TITLE, *A Size That Fits*, means different things to different people. By the time you finish the book, you'll know I'm not referring to the size of your clothes. Instead, I hope you'll find a perfect fit by attaining energy and health based on your values, interests, and personality. In my opinion, you only achieve this when your thoughts and behaviors are synchronized.

The hat on the cover, filled with healthy food and a tennis shoe, represents behavior and choices. You might fill your own hat with different food—including a few not-so-healthy items you learned to eat in moderation. Perhaps you'd add a picture of your dog, paws deep in your hat, to remind you about the important daily discipline of walking him.

The particular image on the cover has a special meaning to me because the fresh food came from our small garden. My family and I planted seeds, watched seedlings turn into vegetables, and enjoyed harvesting and eating them together. This activity created happy memories. Gardening is fun, and vegetables taste better when a family becomes part of the process. The hat on the cover sits atop my daughter's head, with her beautiful eyes below. I pulled the tennis shoe from my son's closet. My mother baked the chicken leg in her oven, and my talented nephew edited the image to make it work on the cover. In short, the cover subtly illustrates why health matters so much to me: My family brings meaning to my life and healthy eating and exercise fit perfectly into enjoying time with them.

Table of Contents

Foreword

WHEN MY FORMER psychology intern David Creel asked me to write a foreword for his upcoming book, I was quite flattered. I've long been impressed with Dave's commitment to the field of obesity, his triple-hitter store of relevant knowledge (nutrition, exercise science, psychology), and his empathic and effective clinical approach in helping his patients draw on his many founts of expertise. A self-help book by someone like him should be a hit!

Unfortunately, once I read the manuscript, I was less happy to be associated with it.

This book will be a failure, a sales disaster, a bullet-train to the remainders pile. Even Amazon won't be able to create a "best-sellers" list long enough to find it.

Why will it fail? Because it violates every tried-and-true rule of weight loss books. It doesn't promise rapid weight loss; in fact it doesn't even *recommend* that. It offers no never-before-revealed secret that will show you how to finally unlock the doors to weight loss, and worse, it subjects the reader to... *facts*. No comforting dismissal of the need for exercise, no easy way to Boost Your Metabolism. It builds no case for a magic food that will help you effortlessly shed pounds, and offers no indictment of some deadly (but common) food that, once eliminated, will put you on the path to success. No testimonials of miraculous cures, no celebrity endorsements, no spinoff products.

Don't even think about a Dr. Oz appearance.

What *does* this book offer? A previously unthinkable combination of weight-control science, clinical experience, compassion, humor, humanness, and humility. Real and relevant scientific information offered in appetizing, usable and bite-sized portions, on a tempting platter of readability and reasonableness. Respect for your intelligence and the multitude of competing demands you face, by the most knowledgeable, unassuming and engaging expert author you could hope for.

Dave (whose warm and approachable demeanor in person is accurately reflected in this book and makes it difficult to call him "Dr. Creel" for more than a page or two) performs a real trick here. He does a wonderful job of presenting what might be dense, eye-glazing scientific information not only in understandable terms, but also in a way that shows he truly appreciates the challenges of incorporating such important information into busy and stressful lives.

You won't find a day-by-day diet; you won't find Barnumesque promises; you won't find a lot of psychobabble; but you will find a storehouse of helpful and relevant solid information, delivered in a way that helps you apply it to your life. This book could be your long-term partner in your efforts to achieve a healthier weight and healthier lifestyle. I will recommend it to colleagues, patients and friends.

Buy it now, read it, and do your best to apply it in your life as needed.

Patrick M. O'Neil, PhD

Past President, The Obesity Society

Director, MUSC Weight Management Center

Professor

Department of Psychiatry and Behavioral Sciences

Medical University of South Carolina

Charleston, South Carolina

Introduction

I WROTE *A Size That Fits* for anyone who's interested in weight loss, and especially for the perpetual dieter. After working with overweight people for over twenty years, I've learned many things about the not-so-obvious aspects of weight management. I now realize that most people already know what to do—or they quickly learn about healthy behavior. Nevertheless, they try diet after diet, feeling worse after each successive failure.

Many of my clients have struggled with weight loss for years. Sometimes they shed pounds on a rigorous diet, buy new clothes, and celebrate victory. But the weight creeps back, along with discouragement and anger at themselves. Their hope quickly fades. They feel weak and sometimes even worthless. How did it happen so fast?

Clinicians know the success rate for treating obesity is low.

The probability of achieving and maintaining a ten percent weight loss without bariatric surgery is about the same as rolling a seven using two dice. That's only a one-in-six chance. But I promise you that losing weight and keeping it off isn't based on luck.

I don't believe people are doomed to obesity. Although losing weight is never easy, I believe each of us has the ability to make permanent changes that result in a healthier weight. We can load the dice by using many different techniques—none of which will land us in jail for a casino-related scheme.

Healthy living doesn't look exactly the same for each person. That's why *A Size That Fits* doesn't promote a one-size-fits-all approach. Instead, it's about the *process* of effectively managing weight. Within these pages, along with ideas for healthy living, you will learn how to let go of unrealistic expectations, learn from your past accomplishments and failures, and become resilient when things don't go as planned.

Instead of a rigid, restrictive diet plan, we'll explore how thoughts, emotions, and past experiences can work in your favor. Stories and patient experiences will help you change your thinking and strengthen specific skills, including:

- maintaining persistence,
- eating mindfully,
- setting goals,
- managing the food environment,
- quieting emotional eating,
- and preventing relapse.

The techniques and ideas in this book are based on important research combined with practical lessons I learned from patients and clients. I don't offer a never-before-told-six-weeks-to-a-slimmer-you plan. Instead, you'll receive a psychological framework to help you lose weight and maintain a new and healthier weight, no matter what kind of reasonable eating style you settle into.

At times you will see me, the author, in these pages, as I share experiences with patients and discuss why I joined the battle against obesity. But this book isn't about me. I want you to find yourself in these pages. As you make healthy changes I hope you'll look beyond numbers on the scale and the tags on your clothing. I encourage you to find a deeper meaning in your endeavors. Personal change is part of living purposefully and can place seemingly unimaginable possibilities within our reach. Like a sunrise that glistens on the surface of the ocean,

I hope *A Size That Fits* will shine healing light into your life and help release your potential to shed poor health and excess weight. Our goal, together, is to achieve permanent weight loss bathed in contentment, confidence, and resiliency. During this journey, you will ponder how your health and weight impacts what matters most to you. By remaining steadfast with this approach, you will discover many things–including a size that fits.

SECTION I

IN THIS SECTION you'll read about how the pleasure of food, our emotions, and the environment can impact food choices and physical activity.

We will explore ways to find pleasure without food, cope with life's problems in healthy ways, and modify the environment.

Chapter One

The Author's Journey

THE YEAR WAS 1994. Elvis' daughter Lisa Marie Presley married Michael Jackson. Michael Jordan played professional baseball and OJ Simpson was arrested for a double homicide of his ex-wife and her male friend. The Eagles finally reunited for a tour and *Forrest Gump* was a must-see movie for about $4.00 a ticket.

As a 25-year-old master's degree student studying clinical exercise physiology at Indiana University, I had already completed clinical nutrition training and proudly added the letters R.D. to my name as a registered dietitian. I also had an undergraduate degree in exercise science. Muscle physiology, macronutrients, the origins of rutabaga—everything was still fresh in my mind.

Brimming with ivory-tower confidence, I felt well equipped to share my knowledge and make the world a healthier place. I found the science of obesity intriguing during my undergraduate training and enjoyed working with people who were overweight. Now I would hone my skills as a weight management counselor by working in a fitness clinic that provided weight loss services for people who wanted to lose 20 to 40 pounds. I enjoyed the clinic's relaxed environment and could hardly wait to begin meeting clients.

However, a woman named Brenda would soon reveal the mismatch between my confidence and my abilities. She came into the clinic looking for help with her weight and I, with my dual training and interests, seemed the perfect counselor.

"Hi, are you Dave?" she asked softly as our paths crossed in the clinic lobby. Before I could finish my reply, she nervously interrupted, "The lady down the hall said it was okay to stop in without an appointment. She said I could probably catch you before you went home."

"I imagine you spoke to our office manager," I said as I picked up a magazine from a chair and placed it back in the rack. "I'm just getting ready to lock up and turn off the lights—you got here just in time!"

"Oh, should I come back later?"

"No, no. I was planning on studying in the back office for quite a while. How can I help?"

On this cool, rainy day, Brenda wore a khaki green trench coat that seemed a bit too long. Her face was flushed because of the long walk to the building, or perhaps because of the uncomfortable topic she needed to discuss. She politely reached out her hand. "I'm Brenda."

"It's nice to meet you," I said, stepping back enough to respect her personal space but close enough to hear her quiet voice.

Standing close, her size was less obvious; I noticed her deep-set blue eyes and long eyelashes. I also noticed sweat running down her face and dripping off the tip of her freckled nose. Perspiration on her neck matted her strawberry blonde, shoulder-length hair as she began telling me she needed help controlling her weight.

As we talked in the lobby, I realized Brenda already knew a lot about nutrition and healthy eating. She told me she enjoyed exercise. Even though she never told me her weight, Brenda was the heaviest person I'd met in a professional setting.

I couldn't tell Brenda, "I know exactly how you feel," because I had never been overweight. But dieting was familiar to me because I was a former high-school and collegiate wrestler. Although my experiences were less extreme than many wrestlers, I knew what it was like to restrict food, deny myself when I was hungry, and cross my fingers when I stepped on the scale trying to "make weight." These experiences with wrestling sparked an early interest in nutrition and exercise.

My desire to help people probably evolved from my upbringing as a pastor's kid, which gave me a heart for people who were often marginalized by the medical community and stigmatized or ignored by others. The work felt purposeful and most of my overweight clients in the clinic seemed appreciative and kind. Although I had great passion and a strong desire to help people, my skills were raw and I often oversimplified my clients' weight-related challenges. This approach made me overestimate my ability to help people change.

During that initial conversation with Brenda, I wondered how I could help her. She seemed intelligent and already understood nutrition, meal planning, and exercise. Yet, with all her knowledge, Brenda was at least 200 pounds overweight. What could I offer? Not my usual nutrition advice and low-calorie recipes. I needed time to think. Knowing I wanted to help Brenda, but not give her false hope, I stalled.

"Let me take your coat. If you'd like, I can tell you a little bit about the services we offer here."

But I knew that *our* services would primarily be *my* services if she joined the program. As the only registered dietitian on staff, I would be helping her lose weight. Although she could attend some of our fitness classes, Brenda and I would partner in her weight loss efforts: I didn't want to disappoint her. After hanging up her coat I offered her something to drink and took my time at the water cooler while she waited in the consultation room. I told myself that even if I couldn't help her, I could listen, let her know I cared, and do my best to find a suitable treatment plan.

When our conversation resumed, Brenda cooled off and I calmed down. I told her about my training and experience and she seemed to sense my genuine desire to help. At that point I had serious doubts about my abilities, but Brenda believed I could help her. In retrospect, she probably felt relieved to hear our program would be relatively straightforward— we would set goals to eat differently and exercise more. We had no discussion about examining her relationship with food, overcoming emotional barriers to success, or using psychological principles to change behavior. I still hadn't refined my skills in those areas. Nevertheless, our personalities seemed to mesh and we agreed to work together.

In our first session I wanted to assess her weight history and eating habits. I still recall how she answered my question about how she gained weight.

"I have poor eating habits—I make bad choices," she said. With her psychological defenses held high, she didn't offer the details I hoped for and needed.

The food journal I asked her to keep didn't help either. She reported eating a fairly healthy diet. She enjoyed vegetables and fruit and often got protein from beans, tofu or other soy products. Despite her reports of balanced eating and portion control, she didn't lose weight. I knew something was missing.

As we continued working together she became more comfortable and remained consistent with her appointments. She attended our fitness classes and became friends with other clinic members and staff. We all found Brenda to be kind and fun-loving, often taking part in practical jokes carried out on the exercise leaders. If one of the muscle-bound instructors walked around in pink socks, we all knew Brenda probably had something to do with his pre-class, gym-bag switcheroo. During individual sessions, Brenda told me a lot about her past experiences and current interests. But when the subject turned to eating and lack of weight loss, she always became vague. I suspected she didn't want to lie, yet wasn't ready to tell me what was really going on.

Over several months of exercise sessions and nutrition counseling, she disclosed small pieces of a childhood filled with abuse and abandonment. Despite her willingness to share her painful past, she still wouldn't reveal her eating patterns. Only near the end of treatment did I begin to glimpse behind the veil and see frequent binge eating, the shame she felt, and the feelings of hopelessness about her weight.

Although I knew enough to refer Brenda to a mental health professional, I didn't have the skills to help her the way I had hoped. I didn't ask the right questions, and I don't know what I would have done if she answered those questions.

Brenda was a stress eater who needed to learn how to manage her emotions differently. How could I help her handle guilt, shame, and the tendency to hide what she was doing? Her therapist helped, but I found it difficult to pull together the concepts she discussed in therapy with the behaviors she and I worked on together. Maybe the best diet counselor on the planet couldn't have helped Brenda lose weight at that time in her life. I don't know. But I realized I had a lot to learn and needed to develop more skills in order to help people like Brenda.

She taught me that effectively treating obesity went far beyond telling people how to eat and exercise. Weight loss is often a personal and painful battle that can't be won through diet education or exercise instruction alone. No matter how much I knew about metabolism, calories, or the nutrients in foods, I couldn't help people who already knew what to do but were psychologically ill-equipped to take action.

Soon after working with Brenda, with a master's degree in hand, I moved away from the familiar confines of a college town and accepted my first job that would pay the rent without a roommate. My new position as a health educator included leading weight management groups and providing one-on-one nutrition and exercise counseling. Several years later I accepted a position at a medical-center-based weight management program. As the program director, I not only had the chance to design and implement treatment, but also learned a great deal from the multidisciplinary team we assembled. I especially enjoyed learning from our psychologist John Guare, who was trained in the obesity field and had a wonderful knack for working with patients.

John and I often discussed how to address issues that derailed our patients. I intently watched him coach people through difficult situations. What did he suggest for the seemingly unmotivated patients, or the ones who lapsed when their lives became stressful? How did he help patients like Brenda who already knew what to do but had layers of psychological obstacles?

John was gracious with his time. His compassionate approach piqued my interest to learn more, and dozens of patients left me searching for more knowledge, skills, and effective approaches to treat obesity. Four years after my work with Brenda, a personal hardship nudged me to fully commit to the training I longed for.

A Lesson in Empathy

We had a rough winter that year, but the promise of spring brought longer days and slightly warmer weather. Evenings remained chilly and the drafty windows on the main floor of my nearly 100-year-old house made the rooms uncomfortable, so I headed upstairs to turn in earlier than usual. I felt tired; at least that's what I told myself, knowing the situation wasn't that simple. As I walked up to my room, the creaky wooden stairs moaned with each step. My short-lived marriage and subsequent divorce left my house feeling barren, uninviting, and cold. Every sound seemed to echo in unwelcomed silence. The house felt abandoned—and so did I. But another long day had finally ended. After a little reading in bed, the cold, empty feelings gave way to sleep. Later, I began to dream.

In a vivid, fairy-tale scenario I found myself swaying back and forth on an old wooden swing in an isolated countryside. The swing's rope connected to the thick branch of an oak tree, but this was not a friendly child's swing. I dangled 30 or 40 feet above the ground, alone in the middle of nowhere. Not knowing how I got on the swing, worry filled my mind as I sat suspended far above the earth below. How would I ever get down? Jumping would probably kill me, and I was afraid to try climbing the ropes because the slightest movement rocked me back and forth. The swing kept rocking as I gazed straight ahead, paralyzed by fear. After a while, I gripped the rope and closed my eyes in despair. I wouldn't open my eyes or look down, knowing this would only remind me of my plight. But a hint of logic finally squeezed through my fear and I mustered the courage to gaze at the reality below. It required the same sort of courage as a child who, fearful of the dark, finally pops his head out from underneath the covers.

To my surprise, the ground was now right below my feet. I could easily step off the swing and walk away. Puzzled and confused, I cautiously closed my eyes and reopened them to confirm what I'd seen. When I opened my eyes, my body began to relax as I fully realized I was safe. I paused again, furrowing my brow and gently biting the inside of my cheek. Had I seen things wrong the first time? Did swinging cause the rope to stretch?

As I stepped off the swing into thick green grass, I took a deep, refreshing breath and turned to look behind me. Like a roller coaster ride with one last unexpected drop, my heart raced and my head filled with wonder. I wasn't alone after all. The landscape was filled with people who had fear and loneliness in their eyes, not realizing they too were swinging only a few feet off the ground.

I've never made much of dreams and often dismiss their significance, knowing that a television show, a passing comment from a co-worker, or a late-night snack can be to blame. But this dream whispered hope and encouragement like no other dream I remember. Although my divorce didn't seem fair, it happened. Up to that point in my life, things had gone pretty well. I had experienced few injustices and often received blessings I felt I truly didn't deserve. Now things were different and I had a choice. I could let anger, loneliness, and distrust turn me into a bitter person; or I could use my experience to help others. Although I didn't like my lesson in empathy, I now had the capacity to better understand the blanket of negative thoughts and emotions that envelop people when life experiences don't match our hopes and expectations. I wasn't alone, and my hardship could serve a purpose. The people on the swings were like me, and though their problems may have been far worse than mine, each of them needed encouragement to look down, step off the swing, and fully embrace life.

Not long after that I applied to PhD programs in clinical psychology. I wanted to better understand human behavior, knowing this would enhance my ability to help people who were overweight. I was accepted by Louisiana State University where, along with a premier football program, they have a world-renowned obesity-related research center. The Pennington Biomedical Research Center seemed like the Obesity Research Hall of Fame to me. During the previous ten years, I read seminal papers about various aspects of obesity. Now, many of the researchers I admired had offices just down the hallway. In addition to required coursework, my clinical training focused on obesity and eating disorders—exactly what I needed to complement my skills. I am grateful for those mentors, friends, and my current wife who was adventurous enough to marry me while in school and help me along the way.

After completing my training at LSU and a one-year internship at the Medical University of South Carolina, where again I focused on working with overweight clients, I returned to Indiana where I still live with my wife and our children. I'm in my second decade of work at St. Vincent Bariatrics, which has one of the largest bariatric surgery programs in the country. In addition to surgical services, our center provides nonsurgical weight management programs for adults and children.

Just as I learned so much from Brenda, I still learn from patients as I carry out nutrition, exercise, and psychology-based interventions to help them lose weight and improve their quality of life. I'm also fortunate to be an active member of a research team, where I mostly focus on promoting physical activity among people who are overweight.

Chapter 2

Missing the Forest for the Peas: Finding the Right Weight Loss Plan

THIS BOOK IS focused on finding the right weight for *you*. Alas, I can't give you a magic bullet to make weight drop off without any effort on your part. Reaching your healthy weight does include nutritious eating and regular physical activity — but I don't want you to become derailed by debatable and impractical advice about dieting and exercise.

Chronic dieters often develop a rigid, perfectionistic mindset while trying to lose weight. Why? Because this works — in the short run. They follow a plan, whatever it might be, until they can't follow it any longer, and then revert back to old eating habits and regain weight. I'll never forget the wife of one of my patients who called the office to complain about her husband Greg. He did well following the advice we outlined and lost a lot of weight. Early in the program we encouraged him to weigh and measure his portions. Unbeknownst to our staff, Greg took portion control to another level — each morning he was literally counting his Cheerios!

Yes, it's important to have structure, personal discipline, and routines while losing weight. But the weight program shouldn't take over your entire life. We can transform our lifestyles when we learn to be flexible, not rigid, in our approach to nutrition and physical activity. Going to extremes as Greg did makes it hard for you to maintain — and enjoy — your new way of living.

> *We can transform our lifestyles when we learn to be flexible, not rigid, in our approach to nutrition and physical activity.*

In this chapter I highlight important points to help you set realistic expectations and achievable goals. I will not give you a specific diet and exercise program to follow. Instead, I offer the tools you need to select a program that's a perfect fit for you.

The biggest issue with weight loss isn't lack of information. The problem lies in sorting through all the diet/exercise plans, books, web sites, blogs, and commercial programs to figure out what works and what doesn't. Another issue with so much information is that the overall message is confusing. Every internet search, news story, or interaction with friends seems to provide advice that contradicts what we thought we already knew.

Rather than add to the confusion, I want to share the nutrition and exercise principles I believe matter most. You don't need to be a nutrition or fitness expert to successfully manage your weight, but basic knowledge will help keep you on track. When I mention *healthy eating* or *regular exercise* later in the book, you can refer to this chapter as a reminder of what those terms mean.

What I'm about to write may fly in the face of things you've read or tried. It may even make a few of you angry. Bananas are not at the root of the obesity epidemic; carrots are not going to throw you into a tailspin of diabetes and heart disease; and peas, yes peas, are an acceptable vegetable. Let me take it one step further: Potatoes can be part of a diet that helps you lose weight, and if you want a diet soda now and then, be my guest.

If you're already worked up, don't start your hate mail yet; gluten-free and organic aren't the panacea for all that ails you, and a debate between low carb and low fat isn't worth our time. If you disagree that's fine. Don't feel obligated to eat bananas, bread, peas, or potatoes. If you believe artificial sweeteners make you crave sweets or cause chronic disease, no need to include them in your diet. If you subscribe to a lower carbohydrate or gluten-free diet, we can find enough common ground to develop a plan that works. But when we get overly caught up in certain aspects of nutrition or weight management, we sometimes end up missing the big picture. If you avoid eating vegetables and fruits because organic isn't available or you can't afford it, you're not doing yourself any favors. If you like mainly starchy vegetables but avoid them because of calories, I encourage you to rethink your plan. If avoiding carbs leads you to choose hot dogs over peaches, that may not be the best choice.

Calories In, Calories Out

If I asked you to tell me in simple terms why someone is in debt, what would you say? Admittedly, finances can be complicated, but let's cut to the core of it: people are in debt because they spend more money than they earn. They may spend too much, earn too little, or both.

By comparison, obesity is also a complex condition we can explain in simple terms. We gain weight when we absorb more calories than we burn. We lose weight when expend more calories than we consume. Like debt, many factors influence the calories-in-calories-out equation. Our genetics are certainly a factor, but rarely can we isolate one gene that makes us gain weight. Instead, a combination of genes may impact our physiology and our response to obesity-promoting environments. Even the bacteria in our guts may influence appetite or how efficiently we use the calories we consume.

Although not likely, it's possible to lose weight eating doughnuts for breakfast, white-bread bologna sandwiches for lunch, and ice cream for dinner. As long as the calories you absorb from these foods are less than the calories burned, you, and your not-so-happy digestive and circulatory systems, will lose weight. That's one reason the discussion about which diet is best (Atkins, Paleo, SouthBeach, Zone etc.) isn't so important. Calories matter more than the source of those calories.

> *Calories matter more than the source of those calories.*

A multi-site study published in the *New England Journal of Medicine* showed that two-year weight loss did not differ among people who followed four different reduced-calorie diets. Over 800 subjects were randomly assigned to eat one of the following:

- a low-fat/average protein diet,
- a low-fat/high protein diet,
- a high-fat/average protein diet,
- or a high-fat/high protein diet.

Their carbohydrate intake was 35 to 65 percent of the calories they consumed, depending on the combination of fat and protein. Each participant's diet was set 750 calories below what he or she needed to maintain weight at the beginning of the study. Not only was weight loss similar between groups, their hunger and levels of satisfaction were the same with each diet.

These results, along with other studies, suggest there is no single, optimal diet for weight loss. This is great news for people who want to lose weight, because you can choose from a variety of nutritional practices, based on your own preferences and lifestyle. Here's the most important question to ask:

Is the reduced-calorie diet I want to follow both healthy and sustainable?

If your answer is, "yes," then I encourage you not to call it a *diet*. Being on a diet sounds like a short-term project. Instead, I hope you'll learn to eat in a way you can continue for the rest of your life. Think of it as your *eating style*.

The Calorie Gallery

Calories are simply units of energy, related to the amount of heat given off when we burn a food. If you want to test this, set a bag of cheese puffs on fire and compare it to the flame you get when you try to light raw broccoli. The orange little logs will burn and give off heat because they are high in calories coming primarily from fat. The broccoli is mostly water, has few calories and definitely won't stoke your campfire.

When you expend approximately 3500 more calories than you absorb, you lose about 1 pound. There are exceptions to this, especially early in the weight loss process when you lose weight more quickly than this equation predicts. That's because when we first begin losing weight, fluid losses accompany the use of small amounts of stored carbohydrate in the muscle and liver. You may also find you lose a few pounds during a hard workout. Even though you only burned several hundred calories, you perspired a great deal and lost water weight you'll regain after rehydrating.

A typical man burns approximately 2500 calories per day and an average woman burns about 2000 calories per day — sorry, ladies. Our energy needs are based on how many calories we burn at rest (our resting metabolism) plus the calories we burn while moving around throughout the day. Resting metabolism is primarily related to the amount of muscle we have. Since men tend to have more muscle than women they, on average, burn more calories. As we unintentionally gain excess weight, muscle is commonly up to 25% of that weight. Therefore, people who are overweight usually burn more calories at rest than those who are not. Generally speaking, the more we weigh, the more calories we burn. As we lose weight, we burn fewer calories unless we increase our physical activity.

Without knowing your weight and level of activity, I can't tell you exactly how many calories to consume in order to lose weight. However, a 1500 to 2000 calorie meal plan is generally appropriate for women, while 2000 to 2500 calories usually results in weight loss for overweight men. If you have fewer pounds to lose, you may need to focus on the lower ends of these ranges, whereas if you are heavier (and burn more calories), you will probably lose weight at the upper ends of these ranges.

I commonly hear from patients, "I can't lose weight eating *that many* calories." What I've found, and research supports, is that most people significantly underestimate the calories they consume. Plus, as I mentioned above, the simple formula of calories in/out, is a dynamic equation. As we lose weight, our bodies progressively require fewer calories for resting or activity. Unless we further drop our calorie intake or increase physical activity, weight loss will slow and eventually stop. Although this is a great mechanism to help prevent starvation, it's frustrating when you expect continued weight loss while following the same plan.

Table 1 shows that dietary calories come from four primary sources: carbohydrate, protein, fat and alcohol.

Calorie Source	Examples	Calorie Density
Carbohydrates	Rice, pasta, bread, cereal, potatoes, fruit, table sugar	4 calories per gram
Protein	Eggs, beef, fish, chicken, pork, beans, dairy	4 calories per gram
Fat	Nuts, oils, seeds, dairy, meats, many processed foods	9 calories per gram
Alcohol	Beer, wine, whiskey	7 calories per gram

You can see from the above macronutrients that fat is the most calorie-dense, at 9 calories per gram of fat. From a calorie perspective, a little fat goes a long way. If you eat a high-fat diet, portion control is of the utmost importance. Imagine you're deciding between eating pork sausage or baked cod for dinner. Three ounces of fat-laden sausage contains about 300 calories, compared to 100 calories for the same amount of the almost fat-free fish.

Getting Practical

Researchers have demonstrated the benefits of low carbohydrate, low fat, low glycemic index, high protein, Mediterranean, and vegetarian diets. People who follow these diets are often passionate about the superiority of one over another. I've discovered that even the most well-informed people can take opposing views of the same data. I once observed two respected scientists vehemently arguing during a symposium related to glycemic index and weight loss. One believed his data clearly demonstrated that glycemic index is important for health and weight regulation. The other professor argued that, because of study design and poor control over other dietary variables, glycemic index by itself is not a crucial component of health and weight. (Glycemic index is basically a measure of how much a food will raise your blood sugar after you eat it).

The tone of this debate reminded me of the guys from *The Big Bang Theory* turning into professional wrestlers. As the presenters debated, I felt more entertained than educated. My mind wandered. I imagined a crowd of screaming academic fans showing up for the Glycemic Index Smack-Down between these two cerebral powers. In this case the fans, including me, were cheering for their respective nutrition star while taking notes and checking references on their mobile devices. The presenters, with sweaty, not-so-beefed-up bodies, took turns grabbing the microphone from the moderator and shouting about insulin response and visceral fat accretion.

"You see these (pointing to his below-average sized biceps)? Believe me, these didn't come from mashed potatoes or skinny little sucrose-laden carrots!"

The debate was interesting, but as a clinician I knew it didn't matter much to most of my patients. I don't want to minimize anyone's work because understanding principles of nutrition at a basic level can guide our recommendations. But for many of my clients, focusing on the glycemic index of vegetables is like having a discussion about updating the hardware on their kitchen cabinets after the roof has blown off the house.

Although people who lose weight in a healthy way and keep it off don't eat exactly the same way, we know that eating within a certain framework will promote health and increase your likelihood of success. The following recommendations are consistent with The Dietary Guidelines for Healthy Americans. You can safely follow these guidelines to lose weight and keep it off in a healthy manner. Of course, if you have a medical condition that requires a special diet, you should consult a registered dietitian. If you've undergone bariatric surgery your guidelines will be somewhat different, especially in the early months after surgery.

Eat Foods from Each Food Group

Over the past 60 years The United States Department of Agriculture has promoted healthy eating through The Basic Four Food Groups, The Food Guide Pyramid, MyPyramid and MyPlate. Even though the recommendations change slightly over time, research continues to support the importance of eating a variety of foods from different food groups. In order to avoid malnutrition, people either have to eat this way or take supplements. Although supplements can play a role in our health, especially for people who have malabsorption issues, food allergies, or intolerances, relying on supplements for health and nutrition isn't ideal.

Scientists are still discovering compounds in foods that may help prevent diseases such as cancer and heart disease. Since we still don't know how all of this works, we can't simply pull out all the beneficial compounds in foods and put them into a pill. For instance, fruits and vegetables contain many phytochemicals (plant chemicals) that play a role in preventing cell damage or assist in health-promoting enzymatic reactions. A typical multivitamin doesn't contain these phytochemicals. Frozen pizza, chicken nuggets, and a handful of supplements are not equal to a diet rich in vegetables, fruit, lean protein sources, whole grains, and low-fat dairy. When we eat selections from all the food groups we naturally maintain a reasonable balance between protein, carbohydrate and fat, and we're likely to consume adequate amounts of vitamins and minerals. People who undergo bariatric surgery are an exception and require vitamin/mineral supplementation.

Eat Different Kinds of Vegetables, and Lots of Them

Eating a variety of vegetables is not only good for you; it also makes weight management easier. Vegetables, especially the non-starchy ones, are mostly water. Chewing these water-filled, nutrition giants will help you feel satisfied on fewer calories. Suppose you're having a turkey sandwich for lunch and decided to have a two-ounce bag of potato chips along with it. The chips contain about 300 calories and 20 grams of fat. If instead you chose to eat raw cauliflower, you could eat two small heads, or about 100 florets, for 300 calories. Of course you'd end up eating much less than that, and therefore consume fewer calories.

Ditch the Sugar-Sweetened Beverages

This is easier said than done for many people. I'm not generally one to promote absolutes when it comes to diet. In fact, I often try to help patients eat problem foods in moderation rather than avoid them altogether. But for the person who drinks multiple regular sodas every day and describes it as an addiction, abstinence is probably the best goal. Why the different approaches with food versus drinks? The healthfulness and allure of most sugar-containing foods vary a great deal. For instance, if someone tells me he's "addicted to sweets," I don't really know what that means. Anything with sugar, like canned corn and pickled beets? Is a graham cracker a sweet, or how about a macaroon? You get the point. With drinks, the categories are easier. Either it's a regular soda or it's not.

People who regularly drink sugar-sweetened beverages often follow patterns like people with addictions, such as smoking. A smoker may always smoke at certain times of day, and soda drinkers often have similar patterns they find hard to break. Studies suggest that regularly consuming sugar-sweetened beverages probably doesn't impact everyone's weight in the same way. The people most likely to gain weight are those with a genetic predisposition for obesity. If you have certain obesity promoting genes (many different genes influence body weight), it's a bad idea to regularly drink sugary beverages. You're like a person with a genetic tendency for asthma who lives in a polluted city. Just as it may be best for that person to find a better place to live, you may want to consider avoiding sugar-sweetened drinks. Although water is probably the best replacement, drinking liquids with artificial sweeteners will greatly reduce calories and can help you lose weight.

Eat Your Fruit, Don't Drink It

Fruit is also relatively low in calories and packed with nutrients. Many well-intentioned people drink fruit juice rather than other sugar-sweetened beverages in an attempt to be healthier. Although fruit juice is more nutritious than soda, the calories are about the same. In addition, research is clear that chewing food makes us feel more satiated than drinking those same calories. Let's say you typically feel satisfied after eating a breakfast including two eggs, two slices of toast, and a twelve-ounce glass of orange juice. If you substituted water for orange juice and ate a clementine instead, you could save calories. In fact, you would need to eat five clementines to equal the calories in twelve ounces of orange juice.

Choose Whole Grains

Our bodies like to operate on sugar (glucose), especially when we exercise at high intensities. When we eat whole grains, complex carbohydrates break down and sugar slowly enters our bloodstream, ready for use by our brain and working muscles. Whole grain foods such as wheat bread, brown rice, quinoa, and oats are rich in vitamins and minerals as well as fiber. Whole grains can be slightly higher in calories, which you will see if you compare white bread to whole wheat bread, because they contain the germ of the seed—a source of healthy fat. Despite the slightly higher calories, you'll probably feel fuller longer because the whole grain fiber slows the rate at which food empties from the stomach. In addition, many foods made with refined grains (crackers, muffins, pastries, cookies, etc.) have added fats and sugars that boost the calorie count and increase our drive to overeat them.

Eat Lean Protein at Meals and Snacks

Calorie-for-calorie, protein tends to be more satiating than fat or carbohydrates. If I asked you to rate your fullness after eating 300 calories of pasta with red sauce (carbohydrates) versus the same calories worth of cheesecake (a tiny piece loaded with fat), compared to boneless skinless chicken breast (almost entirely protein), which would fill you up the most? Studies show it would be the chicken breast. Protein is important to help us feel satisfied after eating. Thus, adding an egg to your breakfast or a low-fat cheese stick to your afternoon snack may help curb overeating later in the day.

Watch for Hidden Fat

For several summers during college I worked breakfast and lunch room service in a high-end hotel. Each morning, dressed in my white Oxford shirt, black pants, and bow tie, I would grab something quick to eat between orders. Oatmeal was my favorite. I wasn't sure why, but this was the best oatmeal ever. I thought maybe the hotel ordered exotic oats from overseas, which would explain the silky texture and rich flavor. Each morning I scarfed down a bowl or two of what I thought was the healthiest thing I could get my hands on. One morning I happened to enter the kitchen when Ms. B, as we called her, was making a large batch of the good stuff. Ms. B was a sweet black lady from Alabama who called everyone Honey. She seemed to cook from the depths of her soul and her food tasted better because you know she prepared it just for you. I can only imagine she learned to cook from her mother, who learned to cook from *her* mother.

Having family from the South, I knew all about the fat-is-flavor style of cooking. But I couldn't believe my eyes when I walked in on Ms. B mid-oatmeal and saw her pouring a large carton of half-and-half creamer into the oats. I never imagined someone could do that to oatmeal! That day I learned a valuable lesson about hidden fat, especially when dining out. People often underestimate the calories in food because they don't account for added fat, especially when others prepare it. Remember, one gram of fat has nine calories. A teaspoon of butter contains about four grams of fat or 36 calories. A stick of butter has over 800 calories (think cookies), compared to an equally sized banana of around 90 calories.

Follow This Diet

In summary, there is no *best* diet for weight loss and weight loss maintenance. But consuming a diet that's rich in vegetables, lean protein sources, fruits, whole grains, and low-fat dairy will make weight loss more likely and give you the best chance of preventing diet-related diseases. In addition, eating a balanced diet can make you feel more energetic and give you the fuel to exercise consistently.

What about Exercise?

Here's a story I've heard many times.

I hired a trainer I saw once a week for two months. I endured grueling workouts and was pretty faithful about working out on my own several times per week. I felt great, my endurance improved, and I could hold a plank for two minutes. But I only lost two pounds. Six-hundred dollars for two pounds! It doesn't seem fair, nor does it make sense.

I agree this doesn't seem fair. After all, when we work hard we want results. However, if we think about it logically, the results do make sense. Compared to making dietary changes, the short-term weight loss we experience from moderate exercise is modest at best.

> *Compared to making dietary changes, the short-term weight loss we experience from moderate exercise is modest at best.*

Shantell is a good example. She reluctantly told me she drank approximately 12 regular sodas per day. Not counting french fries, she hadn't consumed a vegetable in weeks. She and her kids ate fast food almost every day, and the meals she prepared at home included bologna sandwiches, hot dogs, or fish sticks. She would round out her meals with macaroni and cheese, potato chips, or tortilla chips. Although she didn't eat a large volume of food, her diet needed a major overhaul.

Instead of trying to change everything at once, we focused on simply decreasing her soda consumption.

To my amazement, after our meeting she totally stopped drinking the ten-teaspoons-of sugar-per-can stuff. When she returned a month later, she had lost sixteen pounds. She didn't make other changes in her eating, just the soda. If we assume Shantell consumed the same number of calories she was burning at the time we first met (her weight was stable), any calorie reduction would lead to weight loss. Table 2 illustrates how decreasing her consumption of soda (a total of 1800 calories per day) could lead to almost sixteen pounds of weight loss in a month. Remember, burning 3500 calories more than we absorb equates to one pound of weight loss. So the math makes sense. Although Shantell's diet still needed a lot of work, she was able to lose significant weight with only one change in her diet.

Now let's look at how much exercise Shantell would need to do in order to lose a similar amount of weight. She weighed about 350 pounds, so walking burned more calories for her than for someone who weighed less and walked at the same speed. Think of it this way: The more someone weighs, the more work they do when moving that weight a given distance. For example, walking a mile with a 40-pound backpack requires more calories than walking a mile without it. In addition, because of her excess weight, Shantell's resting metabolism was higher than an average-weight woman. I estimated she burned about two calories per minute simply sitting still. Table 3 shows Shantell would burn approximately 140 net calories per mile and would need to walk about 13 miles per day to burn the same number of calories she saved by not drinking 12 cans of soda. At two miles per hour, that would be almost 6½ hours of walking each day!

If you don't drink 12 sodas per day, this example may seem a little extreme. But even if your extra 500 calories come from late night grazing, you'll find it hard to "undo" those dietary indiscretions with physical activity. The point of these math gymnastics is to demonstrate that burning calories through exercise is generally more difficult than saving calories by eating differently. This is especially true for people who can only exercise at low intensity. An elite runner can burn a lot of calories during an hour of exercise, whereas someone taking a slow walk burns far fewer calories. The runner may cover ten miles during that hour, while the overweight person walks two miles an hour. Many studies back up this principle of diet-versus-exercise for weight loss. We know that, in the short run, exercise doesn't directly cause much weight loss. When we look at the long run, it's an entirely different story.

> *We know that, in the short run, exercise doesn't directly cause much weight loss. When we look at the long run, it's an entirely different story.*

Diet Induced Weight Loss			
Diet Change	Calorie Savings per Day	Calorie Savings per Month	30-Day Weight Loss
Stopped drinking 12 sodas/day	12 sodas x 150 calories each = 1800 calories	1800 calories x 30 days = 54,000 calories	54,000 cals/3500 =15.5 pounds

Walking Time Required to Lose 15.5 pounds in One Month		
Extra Calories Burned/Mile	Miles of Walking to = 1800 Calories	Time required to walk 12.8 miles at 2 mph
200 calories per mile - 60 calories burned at rest = 140 net calories	1800 calories/140 calories per mile = 12.8 miles	12.8 miles @ 2mph = 6.4 hours

In order to understand long-term weight loss success, researchers study people who are good at it. Many studies show that people who lose weight and keep it off are physically active. Data from the National Weight Control Registry and many studies conducted by Dr. John Jakicic at the University of Pittsburgh tell us that exercise is a crucial component in keeping lost weight from reappearing. Although studies vary on exactly how much exercise is necessary to keep weight off, most experts agree that engaging in 250 to 300 minutes of exercise each week will greatly increase your chances for success.

You may wonder why short-term weight loss from exercise tends to be modest, yet exercise is almost a requirement if you want to prevent weight regain. Researchers have not yet conclusively demonstrated *why* exercise is related to long-term success in weight loss. Although exercise, especially resistance training, may help prevent muscle loss and a lowering of metabolic rate that accompanies weight loss, not all studies support this idea. But when we look at the many other benefits of physical activity, we can draw logical conclusions about the long-term benefits of exercise.

- The longer we stick with an exercise routine, the more fit we become. As we become more fit, we're able to increase our exercise intensity for longer periods of time. The more we can do, the more calories we burn. When we're feeling fit, we gravitate toward physically challenging things that burn more calories.

- Exercise improves mood. If we feel less depressed and anxious we're less likely to eat emotionally or be distracted from personal health goals.

- While exercising, we are not sitting in front of the TV. If we aren't sitting in front of the TV, we can't be eating in front of the TV.

- If we invest in our bodies by taking time to do good things for them, we probably don't want to abuse the body with unhealthy eating. That would be like intentionally driving through the mud after a car wash.

- For those who enjoy physical competitions with themselves or others, eating is fuel for those endeavors.

If high octane (healthy food) is available, we use it.

- Feeling accomplished about physical activity can improve confidence in other areas, including wise choices in what and how much we eat.

Exercise is Like Medicine

Excess weight is associated with a number of health problems including:

- Type 2 diabetes
- Heart Disease
- High Blood Pressure
- Cancer
- Stroke
- Osteoarthritis
- Sleep apnea
- Liver and gallbladder disease
- Stroke
- Infertility
- High cholesterol and triglycerides
- Dementia

People often want to lose weight to help treat or prevent these disorders. Most people who take medications for these conditions would prefer not to. I often work with patients who take fifteen or more different medications each day. Remembering to take medications multiple times per day, knowing which ones to take with or without food, and refilling prescriptions becomes a significant inconvenience; it's like having a part-time job. The out-of-pocket costs for these drugs can also be substantial. They wish they could just take one pill for everything, or better yet, not have to take pills at all. Although that may not be entirely realistic, there is a "super pill" that will treat or help prevent many of these conditions.

It is free, has few negative side effects and doesn't require a prescription from your doctor or a trip to the pharmacy. It can be used at any time of the day and you can still operate heavy machinery after taking it. Of course this "super pill" is exercise. Physical activity can:

- Reduce the risk of type 2 diabetes
- Decrease the risk of cardiovascular disease
- Manage blood pressure
- Decrease the risk of some cancers
- Improve sleep
- Prevent or treat anxiety and depression
- Increase good cholesterol and decrease triglycerides
- Prevent osteoporosis
- Decrease the risk of dementia

If you compare the list of conditions related to obesity to the list of benefits from exercise, you'll notice the similarities. Not only does exercise help manage weight in the long term; it treats many disorders related to obesity. Overweight people who exercise will improve their health even if they don't lose weight.

Unfortunately, many people view weight loss as the only reason to get moving, and when they don't lose weight they stop, ignoring all of the other potential benefits. Whether you are underweight, normal weight, or overweight, you'll reap health benefits from becoming physically active.

Diet and Exercise. Anything Else?

Successful tools for weight loss are designed to: 1) decrease the number of calories we consume or 2) increase the calories we burn. Following a reduced calorie eating plan and engaging in physical activity should do the trick. But sometimes our best efforts don't work. That's because a host of metabolic, neurochemical, and psychological factors add to the weight loss challenge and make obesity a difficult condition for healthcare practitioners to treat. You'll read more about this later in the book, but here's a summary:

- People can be genetically inclined to obesity. During the first few years of life, some children overeat foods that taste especially good—and these eating patterns appear to be genetically influenced. Over time, people who are genetically susceptible will gain weight due to the imbalance between calories burned and consumed.

- Another weight loss challenge occurs when neurochemicals within the body act on the appetite center of the brain, making prolonged calorie restriction difficult.

- Some medication used to treat obesity-related conditions (such as insulin for diabetes), also makes it hard to lose weight.

Not only do we face these challenges—we're surrounded by a cultural environment that promotes weight gain and taxes our ability to practice restraint.

Although it isn't a new problem, worldwide rates of obesity have increased dramatically over the past forty years. Researchers have kept up with new weight loss medications and surgical procedures, but these were not without a cost. Some medicines were eventually pulled from pharmacies because of cardiovascular concerns, and some surgeries led to malnutrition and even death. This checkered past left many physicians fearful of treating obesity with newer, aggressive medical interventions. They wonder if the next FDA approved medication will cause heart valve problems or strokes. Will the next bariatric surgery yield short-term weight loss, just like other procedures that have fallen out of favor, but be ineffective or dangerous in the long run?

The good news is that scientists and physicians are well educated and typically smart people. Okay, a few seem to have slipped through the cracks, but overall they learn from mistakes and try not to repeat them. Obesity treatment is evolving and our current medical interventions, considering the risks and benefits, are better now than ever. In twenty years they will most likely be better than today.

Unfortunately, while medical treatment keeps improving, the fast food industry, the abundance of delicious, calorie-laden food, and easy access to these foods add new challenges to people who have even a slight predisposition for becoming overweight. Medical science cannot keep up with our growing obesity problem. Because obesity is such a difficult condition to treat, it makes sense to understand all of the tools available and consider if they're a good fit for your situation.

> *Medical science cannot keep up with our growing obesity problem.*

Bariatric surgery for severe obesity

I have interacted with thousands of patients who were considering bariatric surgery. When we measure success by maintained weight loss, bariatric surgery is by far the most effective treatment for severe obesity. However, because of the risk for complications, this surgery isn't used for people with 20 or 30 pounds to lose. To medically qualify and get insurance coverage for the most effective procedures, patients need to be approximately 100 or more pounds overweight or about 75 pounds overweight with problems such as diabetes, heart disease, high blood pressure, or sleep apnea. From an insurance perspective, the degree of obesity is usually determined by body mass index (BMI)—a simple formula that takes into account your height and weight.

If you want to calculate your BMI, simply type "BMI calculator" into your web browser search engine and enter your numbers. A BMI of 18.5 to 25.0 is considered normal. To qualify for the most aggressive bariatric surgeries you'll probably need a BMI of 35 with certain medical conditions, or 40 without them.

Bariatric surgery is a sacrifice of sorts. Initially, you give up the freedom to eat whatever you want, whenever you want, and as much as you want. Granted, with procedures such as the gastric bypass and sleeve gastrectomy, hunger hormones are impacted and can make these sacrifices less difficult than attempting weight loss without bariatric surgery.

Weight loss medication

Medication can help you stick to a low-calorie eating plan, although you won't find a magic pill that makes you lose weight without eating less food and/or exercising. These drugs come with risks, potential side effects, and interactions with other medications that may limit their safety and effectiveness. No medication yields results similar to bariatric surgery. However, when combined with a diligent effort to eat better and get regular exercise, you can expect up to an extra five percent weight loss compared to people who try losing weight without medication. This is ten more pounds for someone who weighs 200 pounds—and that may help you achieve healthier blood pressure, blood sugar, and cholesterol. The most commonly used weight loss medicines decrease appetite by impacting neurotransmitters, the chemical messengers in the brain. Several of the newer medications are actually a combination of two drugs that work together to decrease appetite. Not everyone feels less hungry when they take weight loss medications and some people find that over time the medications seem to have a diminished effect on appetite.

You and Your Physician

When you decide to lose weight, I encourage you to schedule an appointment with your doctor to discuss medications, bariatric surgery, and even newer modes of obesity treatments such as vagus nerve stimulation or the intragastric balloon.

If your physician makes statements such as "I don't believe in bariatric surgery," or "I won't prescribe weight loss medication," then consider finding a provider who's more open-minded.

You may hear people say that using medication or having bariatric surgery is the easy way out—like you're somehow cheating. That's like telling someone, "It's cheating if you drive twenty miles to work instead of walking." Sounds ridiculous, doesn't it? Like driving a car, medication or surgery may be the most practical vehicle to take you where you want to go.

You can cut down a tree with a handsaw or a chainsaw. Actually, if you worked long and hard enough you could cut down a tree with a butter knife. The chainsaw is more dangerous than hand tools, but also more effective. The more sophisticated and powerful the tool, the more risk for injury. So it is with weight management. The stronger tools give you a higher likelihood for success.

Ultimately, you must still do the work. Whether you have bariatric surgery, take weight loss medications, or lose weight without any medical intervention, you're the one who decides what, when, and how much you eat and exercise. You're the one who packs a healthy lunch instead of ordering out, and then laces up your shoes to take a daily walk.

The rest of this book will equip you with strategies that help you make successful lifestyle changes, no matter what weight-management tools you decide to use.

Chapter 3

It's all About Motivation . . . Or is it?

"IF YOU WANT to lose weight badly enough, you will." This is something people often say to me. Sometimes I even hear it from professionals whose patients are ignoring their instructions. Most often I hear it from patients themselves or frustrated family members. But is it true? Is weight management all about motivation? My short answer is *no*.

Motivation is important. This desire to achieve is the first step of an action plan. Without it we'd be unproductive and unhappy. Motivation helps us schedule job interviews, go on first dates, or sign up for exercise classes. Motivation gets us going.

We definitely need motivation to help us lose weight and keep it off, yet motivation tends to wax and wane. Like a match we strike, it burns out.

> *Motivation tends to wax and wane. Like a match we strike— it burns out. Weight management is about sustaining behavior for years.*

Weight management is about sustaining behavior for years. We need the match, but perseverance calls for lighting something that will burn slowly over time. When we put all our eggs into a motivation basket, we're constantly searching for short-term sparks to get us going. This continual rummaging for inspiration can become tiresome. We eventually become so worn out and overwhelmed that our motivation can morph into its cousin, *desperation*.

In this chapter we'll discuss the difference between motivation and desperation. We'll also look at three other attributes for achieving long-term success: commitment, identity and better habits.

Confusing Motivation with Desperation

When you've failed at weight loss many times, your desire to change can turn into something that seems like motivation but isn't. Loretta's story is a good example.

Loretta showed up 15 minutes late for her psychological evaluation for bariatric surgery. I knew little about her aside from the information in her medical records. In her chart, I found that Loretta weighed well over 400 pounds and had diabetes, sleep apnea, arthritis, and low back pain. She checked the African American box on her intake form and I noticed her address was in the middle of a crime-ridden part of a nearby city. When I met her in the waiting room she rocked backward and then forward while pushing on the arms of the chair in order to get to her feet. She groaned and grimaced with pain while walking with me to my office, barely acknowledging my introduction. She didn't apologize for being late and seemed uninterested in small talk about weather or traffic. After we sat down, I explained the purpose of the required evaluation was to make sure surgery was a good fit for her, and if so, determine what things she could do to best prepare for the operation.

As Loretta began telling me about herself, it was clear our lives were only similar in the sense that we were both raised without much direct influence from other cultures and races. Her urban speech patterns were unlike mine, and her life was riddled by poverty and family members incarcerated or addicted to drugs. She casually admitted to having a drug problem in the not-so-distant past. On the other hand, I grew up in a Mayberry-like small town insulated from most of the problems found in inner cities.

Although I've tried to educate myself about other cultures and interact with people different from me, I can't change the color of my skin or how I grew up. I could not simply, without invitation, step into Loretta's world and understand her life. Our differences were important to her and she didn't want to talk about the thing that was most personal to her—her weight—with someone like me. How could I blame her? After all, it's hard enough to talk about personal struggles with someone who understands where you come from. Revealing these things to a stranger from a different culture and race adds to the difficulty.

I listened intently to Loretta and paid close attention to her body language. Although I tried hard to connect, she spoke to me with distrust, answering my questions with curt frustration. She was holding her cards close to her chest, afraid if I got a glimpse I'd take advantage of her. She feared I would win the game and taunt her with condescending psychobabble. Like many patients in this situation, she probably believed I'd use her words against her when it came to deciding if she was an appropriate candidate for surgery.

My attempts to convince her we were "on the same team" and I wanted to help did not resonate. I had real concerns that her lack of a support system, combined with financial hardships, would cause problems for her after surgery. Would she be able to afford the vitamins she needed to take daily for the rest of her life? When she couldn't use food to cope with life difficulties would she turn to drugs again? Although she couldn't see it, surgery could make her life worse if she wasn't ready and equipped to make the necessary changes. As I continued to probe about how she would manage various aspects of her life after surgery, she stopped me.

"I don't like where this is going."

I put down my pen and stopped taking notes. "What are you concerned about?"

"I want to change my life."

"How do you want your life to be different?" I asked, as our eyes finally connected.

Her expression softened and her eyes welled with tears. Like the small movement from the torque on a lid of a never-opened jar, I could sense something was about to give way. At that moment I didn't notice her body that 30 minutes earlier had fallen into the oversized chair, out of breath from walking to my office. I didn't notice her skin tone or the fullness of her face. Our age difference and dissimilar upbringings were insignificant. I just looked into her eyes and felt the gap between us closing. In a strained, high-pitch voice required to delay an ensuing sob, she quickly exclaimed,

"I can't even wipe my own ass anymore."

I didn't know what to say. There it was, one of the most personal and embarrassing aspects of her life, out in the open. In those few words, she ripped through the veil I'd been tugging at the entire session. But I wasn't ready for it; I could no longer sustain eye contact. It was like I accidently saw her naked and was sorry I embarrassed her. As I felt the weight of her troubles, compassion stole my words. I looked down, nodding my head.

"I can only imagine how that makes you feel," I said, after a long pause.

Her size had robbed her of her dignity. She was angry. As we continued talking, I learned she had been this size for quite some time. She depended on her husband to prepare food and help her dress, bathe, and get into and out of her car. It seemed illogical that up to the point of seeking bariatric surgery, she had done little to change course. How could it be that Loretta, like many other people, hated her situation so much, wanted to change, yet seemingly did nothing about it for so long?

Clearly, Loretta wanted to lose weight. In fact, she told me she'd wanted to lose weight for a very long time. Despite her desire for a different life, I imagine she had misguided family members who said, "When she wants it bad enough, she'll do it."

But Loretta's problem wasn't lack of desire. She had a strong desire to lose weight, but she wasn't motivated: Loretta was desperate. A simple comparison will help explain what I mean.

Imagine you're stranded on an island by yourself. You have sources for food, water, and primitive shelter. You're happy to be alive, but also desperate to leave the island, interact with other humans, and enjoy a hot shower. Month after grueling month you try everything to escape the island—sort of like the old TV show *Gilligan's Island*. After years of failed attempts, you still want to leave, but you've given up hope. Deep down you believe nothing will work—and you're losing motivation. Any new idea to get off the island leads to a half-hearted pursuit before giving up. You're so demoralized that you can no longer tell the difference between good ideas and dead ends—they all seem alike.

This is the point Loretta reached with weight management. Someone told her about bariatric surgery and she felt so desperate she made an appointment. She wanted to lose weight, had many good reasons to change, but wasn't motivated. Our conversation revealed that, to her, bariatric surgery was no different than the grapefruit diet, the cold shower and potato diet, or having her mouth wired shut. In her desperation she hadn't considered how this procedure was different than everything else she had tried.

Because of her perspective, she wasn't ready to do the work required to be successful with bariatric surgery. When we offered to help Loretta prepare for surgery by changing her diet and beginning a modest physical activity program, she seemingly lost interest. Maybe over time she became motivated and pursued help elsewhere. Perhaps she's still on her island—I hope not.

> *Desperation occurs at the intersection of hopelessness and motivation. We want to change but have lost hope.*

Desperation occurs at the intersection of hopelessness and motivation. We want to change, but have lost hope. We consider drastic efforts without truly believing they'll lead to success, and after a while the drive to change begins to fade away.

> *Desperation can rob us of clear thinking and make us vulnerable to things that will harm us, while safer solutions rest quietly within our reach.*

Desperation can lead to motivation, but not always. Desperation can also rob us of clear thinking and make us vulnerable to things that will harm us, while safer solutions rest quietly within our reach. Many times people repeat the old saying: "You have to hit rock bottom before you can change." In other words, life has to get *really* bad before we're desperate enough to make changes. This can be true for weight loss, and sometimes it works, but it only works if someone will help you out of the mire and offer a safe, realistic plan. Even then, you must accept the help, believe in the plan, and do your part to make it happen. Otherwise, desperation usually leads to taking whatever someone will give you and hoping things will miraculously work out.

Motivation is the Starting Point

Motivation is an energizing force that often leads to positive action. We feel motivated when we decide the benefits of change outweigh the costs, and we believe in our ability to succeed.

Motivation is the perfect starting point for change, but it tells us little about whether or not we'll carry through in the long run. Home improvement projects are good examples of this. A couple might say, "Wouldn't it be nice to tear down this wall and open the space next to the kitchen? We can increase the value of our home and have more space for entertaining. Plus, we'll save a bundle if we do the work ourselves."

Some families tackle these projects and complete them. Others begin, realize they're in over their heads, and end up calling a contractor to finish the work. Still other people start a home improvement project, hit a rough patch, and leave it unfinished for years. Some of you may have a similar, seemingly never-ending project in limbo. Maybe you're stuck because the work wasn't as simple or inexpensive as you hoped. Perhaps you ran into mold, termites, or a structural beam behind a wall. Or maybe the stress led to so many arguments with your spouse that you no longer feel like doing the work.

If we compare people who finish projects to those who give up, the results have little to do with their initial motivation. Instead, a good outcome is based on their ability to plan, anticipate obstacles, and have both the skills and mindset to deal with complications.

In many ways, weight management is similar to a house remodel. It requires knowledge, planning, tools, and help from others. Although motivation can lead to the decision to work on your weight, it's often a temporary state that won't carry you through a lifestyle change. With home remodeling the work eventually ends. But weight management is forever. What will help you keep going for a lifetime?

Motivation versus Commitment

People who lose weight and keep it off make a commitment to handle this aspect of their lives. Their commitment arises from motivation, and sometimes from desperation. The idea of commitment is easier to understand when we examine how we use this word:

- We commit to our marriages.
- He's committed to his faith.
- She's committed to her career.
- I'm committed to completing my degree.
- They're committed to getting out of debt.
- I'm committed to my family.

Because commitments are often tied to important parts of our lives, most people only make them after much thought and deliberation. Commitments reach into the future; they continue even when motivation wanes; and they are not defined solely by behavior. That is, you can't tell if someone is committed by a snapshot of what she's doing. Are two people who hold hands committed to each other? Is a man who goes to the gym every morning for two weeks committed to his health? Maybe, or maybe not.

True commitment is linked to determination, even when things aren't going well. The committed couple going through a rough spot in their marriage is more likely to say, "How can we make this work?" instead of, "I don't think this is going to work." When committing to something or someone, we expect to make sacrifices. If we're committed to completing a degree, we may watch less TV and study more. When we commit to raising a family we sacrifice time, energy, and sometimes our sanity (just kidding).

> *We should always build motivating factors into a weight loss plan—and these can be fun.*

Along those same lines, people who succeed at managing their weight are committed to the process of managing their health. Their behavior isn't always perfect and motivation can ebb and flow, yet they keep going. That's why it's important to build motivating factors into a weight management plan—and these can be fun. Training for a 5K race, taking a healthy cooking class, planting a garden, or accepting a step challenge from a group of online friends can be motivating and strengthen your commitment. The longer you continue honoring your commitment, the easier it becomes.

Creating Habits and a New Identity

Researchers Rena Wing and James Hill asked, "What do people who succeed at losing weight and keeping it off have in common?" To answer this question, they invited people who'd lost at least 30 pounds and kept if off for a year or more to join the National Weight Control Registry. Over the last 20 years, along with their colleagues and students, they've published studies to help us learn from those who succeed. One of those studies is related to a mindset that may help us succeed with long-term weight management.

In that study, Dr. Mary L. Klem, provided questionnaires to over 900 people in the registry and assessed how they viewed the effort, attention, and pleasure associated with maintaining a lower weight. On average, the participants kept off about a 60-pound weight loss for almost seven years. They reported it became easier to keep their weight steady as time passed, requiring less effort and attention. And, they said the pleasure of maintaining weight loss did not diminish. Less work and continued satisfaction—who wouldn't like that result?

This study shows how commitment can lead to habits that make it easier for us to maintain new behavior. These new, healthier behaviors usually require less motivation and attention because, well, they're habits!

When you develop habits with intention (that is, on purpose), and merge these behaviors with the most important aspects of your life, they become part of your identity. Imagine you begin riding a bike to work or walking an extra mile every day. Imagine taking the stairs instead of the elevator, which is too crowded anyway. Visualize having a fresh, colorful salad for lunch on most days. Imagine having an occasional half-cup scoop of your favorite sherbet for dessert instead of a nightly bowl of ice-cream with hot fudge sauce. Imagine having your favorite decadent food as a special treat, but not eating it in excess.

Once you and others begin to see these behaviors as part of who you are and what you do, these habits become part of your identity. Just as you might describe yourself as a non-smoker, or pet lover, you also describe yourself as a healthy eater or a regular exerciser. Once this happens you begin to forget old unhealthy behavior patterns and the "new you" eventually becomes the "old you." The new way of viewing yourself becomes part of who you are.

I can't promise this is always easy. Many overweight people find it hard to see themselves as an exerciser or healthy eater because they don't *look fit*. Buying extra-large clothing or looking at yourself in a full-length mirror can trigger negative thinking. Women compare themselves to size 4 fashion models, while guys sometimes look at their favorite athletes and tell themselves, "I'll never get there. No use trying." This attitude stands in the way of creating a new identity, and it definitely influences behavior. In fact, it becomes a vicious, self-fulfilling prophecy.

One of my clients told me about an encounter that shows how appearance, background, and conditions need not define our health identity.

Rob has been overweight for years. He's a guy who loves football, beer, and a casual lifestyle. He's single and works with a group of other men who don't cook or even consider what they eat. As a result, Rob consumes a lot of fast food. In his mind, that's what guys do, and so it became part of his identity. Other parts of his identity, less obvious to his friends, are his diabetes, which requires more insulin with each pound he gains, and his recent diagnosis of high blood pressure. Rob also has a heart for helping others, whether it's taking care of a sick family member, building housing in Haiti, or helping a friend move. In a recent visit to my office he told me about an incident that made an impact on his weight loss efforts.

"Doc, you won't believe what happened to me this week. There's this homeless guy I see almost every day close to my work. He's maybe 50 or so—heck we're probably about the same age. Anyway, he has dirty long dreads and he pushes around a shopping cart with some of his personal items. As far as I know he never really panhandles, but for some reason I just feel bad for him. So the other day I saw him on my way to lunch and decided to pick up something for him to eat, too. I was at Hardee's and after I finished eating, I ordered him a cheeseburger, fries and a Coke. I thought I was doing something nice for the guy, you know? So I drove over to where he hangs out and I rolled down my window and said 'Hey man, come here, I got you some lunch.'

He walked over to my car and I handed the sack through the window. But instead of taking the food and saying thanks, he just looked at the sack and said, 'What'd you buy me?'

I said, 'It's just a burger and fries. Go ahead, take it.'

Then this guy says, 'Man, I don't eat that kind of stuff.'

I was like, 'You mean, you don't want it?'

Then he said, 'Nah man, I got diabetes and my doctor told me that sort of food will kill me. If you want to get me something to eat, go over to McDonald's and get me a salad.'

So here I was sitting in my car, with a homeless guy refusing the food I bought him because it wasn't healthy enough. I couldn't believe it!"

Rob went on to tell me this incident made him think about his own behavior. If a homeless person can make good food choices, surely he could too. It also demonstrated that physical appearance and our surroundings don't need to dictate identity. Rob assumed this man's dirty clothes and unkempt appearance meant he wasn't worried about what he ate.

Similarly, overweight people often find it difficult to view themselves as healthy because of their weight or appearance. Remember, a healthy weight results from healthy behaviors. In most cases it won't lead you to a size four or ripped abs. Healthy people come in different shapes and sizes and I encourage you to let go of "ideal weights." Although weight is related to health, it doesn't define it.

> *Healthy people come in different shapes and sizes and I encourage you to let go of "ideal weights." Although weight is related to health, it doesn't define it.*

It's also crucial to accept that our size is only one component of appearance, and appearance is only one small part of who we are. Our intellect, personality, interests, abilities, purpose and pursuits need not be overshadowed by weight. Instead, if our drive for a healthier weight is integrated into other meaningful aspects of our lives, our weight management efforts won't feel like a project disconnected from who we are. If I view managing my weight as part of becoming a better parent because I can go bike riding with my child, then managing weight takes on new meaning. If faith is a driving force in your life that encourages you to help others, your weight and health choices can either help or hinder your efforts.

Finding time to exercise doesn't need to take away from what we give to our careers and the people we love. On the contrary, it will help us think more clearly, work more efficiently, manage stress better, and probably increase our productivity.

Chapter 4

Pay Attention!

AS WE GO through daily life, multiple thoughts enter our heads like a parade that never ends. Each thought may lead to an action that can trigger more thoughts, more behavior, and so on. Our minds relentlessly create judgment, worries, memories, and ideas. For those of us concerned about weight, these thoughts are often related to eating. Like a game of tennis played on the court of life, our thoughts and behaviors are constantly in flux, moving us toward or away from healthy places. When it comes to food, the back and forth of our tennis match may go something like this:

It's nine p.m. and you just finished watching your favorite TV show. Now the food commercials start. In less than 30 seconds you see a woman seemingly transformed by a bite of creamy Greek yogurt. Her eyes close and her head tilts slightly to the side as her lips close softly around this magical spoonful of raspberry swirled yogurt. "Wow, that looks great," you think. You respond to that thought by heading to the refrigerator. You pull the door open and see yogurt, some cheese sticks, and, oh—there's the chocolate sauce. Seeing chocolate sauce reminds you of ice cream in the freezer. Perhaps you should make sure it's there.

Yep, you still have ice cream. You open up the container and consider "cleaning up" the ice cream stuck to the inside edges of the carton and then scraping and tasting until all is symmetrical and level. Should you scoop some into a bowl?

If you decide to eat ice cream, your beliefs about that behavior also have a lot to do with *how much* you eat. Thinking about the flavor instead of the health effects of ice cream can lead to overeating.

Over time, strings of behavior and thoughts like the ones above can lead to bad habits. It's like we're stuck playing tennis on one part of the court. Upcoming chapters will help you learn to change your environment and alter your thinking, but the first step to interrupting these thoughts and breaking bad habits is to pay closer attention to what you're doing.

> *The first step to interrupting thoughts and breaking bad habits is to pay closer attention to what you're doing.*

In the last chapter we discussed motivation and the idea of committing to the process of weight management. This commitment is not simply about how we think—we also commit to taking action, because actions propel us to improve our health and transform our bodies. More importantly, some practices eventually shape our perspectives and become part of who we are.

As a young man, I learned a valuable lesson about dangerous patterns of thoughts and behavior—a lesson that would eventually help me break the risky and costly habit of speeding. At two different times in my 20s, I received multiple traffic tickets within a year. Not only did it cost me money I didn't have to spare, it earned me two separate trips to defensive driving school. If you've never attended a defensive driving class, take my word, it isn't a great way to spend Tuesday evenings. After my second set of enthralling group interactions, I decided I didn't really like the idea of paying fines and watching videos about the dangers of speeding. But speeding was sort of a habit with me. I told myself I was driving with the flow, but in reality I drove with the flow in the far left lane. To avoid getting additional traffic tickets I did two simple things: I noticed the speed limit wherever I was driving, and I frequently checked my speedometer. I stopped "going with the flow." I began paying attention.

"Going with the flow" is one way of describing ingrained habits for eating and exercise. We need to pay attention in order to change eating and activity levels. It may seem you don't eat differently than other people, and that may be true, depending on who you compare yourself to. But if you're gaining weight, or maintaining excess weight, then going with the flow probably won't lead to weight loss.

A Food Diary—Your Ticket to Success

Creating and maintaining a food diary is one of the best ways to increase awareness of what you're doing. A food journal is to an overweight person as a speedometer is to a speed demon trying to slow down.

If you dread the idea of having a paper journal you must pull out each time you eat, hide for fear someone might look at, or misplace multiple times a day, you can relax and let technology eliminate these barriers. A multitude of apps allow us to discreetly track eating and physical activity. It's as simple as pulling out your phone and entering a little information each time you eat. Many of the applications have features that allow you to scan the UPC code of a food in order to add it to your diary. At all times during the day you can see how many calories you've eaten and how many remain, which will guide you during situations like that late-night trip to the refrigerator. You can also pay attention to other dietary factors such as percent of calories coming from fat, protein and carbohydrate, the grams of fiber you have consumed, and so on. If you aren't into technology, there's no reason you can't keep a paper food journal. Many of my patients prefer this simple pen-and-paper method. If you're working with a professional to manage your weight, a food journal highlights the strengths and weaknesses of your diet, and can guide the discussion about your eating patterns.

Tracking food intake will help you pay attention to what you're eating, educate you on the source of calories, allow you to examine patterns of behavior you may want to modify, and help explain why your weight is changing. Whether you use a paper journal, an app, or a website to track your eating, the following suggestions will help you get the most out of self-monitoring.

Include everything you eat

The primary goal of keeping a record is to increase awareness and ultimately change your behavior. Therefore, you should "partner" with your journal, agreeing to report everything you eat. That includes a handful of peanuts, a small piece of candy, a bite of your spouse's cake, etc. Having incomplete or inaccurate food records will frustrate you, because according to the records, you *should* be losing weight, but aren't. Yes, it's a bit inconvenient to record every little thing you put in your mouth, but therein lies the beauty of self-monitoring. It can cause you to pause and ask yourself, "Do I really want these peanuts if I have to record them? Am I really that hungry?" If you're eating out of habit, your food journal is a deterrent to mindless eating and grazing.

Include all beverages containing calories

Many people who record their intake are lackadaisical about including beverages. Soda, juices, alcohol, sport drinks, and even some diet beverages contain calories and can be a significant contributor to weight.

Measure your portions

Although researchers have developed a way to determine portion sizes by taking photos of our food, there is currently no good, commercially available technology to track portion sizes without some work on your part. Weighing and measuring food can be helpful because our eyes fool us into believing we're eating less than we really consume. Although a food label may list ¾ cup of cereal as a serving, that may not be typical for you. Once you determine how much a cup of milk fills your glasses, what one cup of pasta looks like on your plates, and the size of three ounces of meat (about the size of a deck of cards), you may not need to get the measuring cups and food scale out for each meal. However, spot-checking portion sizes is generally a good idea to make sure your perception isn't drifting. If you aren't losing weight as expected, returning to exact measuring may be helpful.

Include the good days and the not-so-good days

We often learn more from our struggles in life than we learn from success. Although it's psychologically challenging to record food intake when we feel as if we're going off the rails, this can be immensely helpful. Tracking deviations helps reveal our relationship with food. Behavior is easier to correct when we're aware of food-related triggers and typical responses. For example, perhaps you overeat when dining out with friends or after a stressful day at work when you feel too tired to cook. People who pay attention to these trigger events usually get off track less often and stay off track for shorter periods, compared to those who feel discouraged, stop being mindful, and abandon the food journal.

Food journaling is part of a larger process of changing your relationship with food. In order to get the most out of it, you need to reinforce healthy behavior, but also understand and change your unhealthy responses to stressful situations.

Record as you go

Record the foods you eat *as you eat them*. Waiting until the end of the day to write down what you're doing is like waiting until you get your credit card statement to determine if you're sticking to a budget. Tracking as you go leads to awareness. You are self-monitoring your behavior rather than just producing a record. In addition, the longer you wait to record your intake, the more you misremember what and how much you ate. It's easy to forget exactly what you consumed, and portion sizes tend to shrink when you rely on memory.

Tell a story

Your food journal should tell a story. When you're losing weight it should be evident why this is occurring. Remember, it takes approximately a 3,500-calorie deficit to yield a pound of weight loss, so we aren't looking at food records to explain day-to-day changes in weight. Rather, we can examine eating patterns over several weeks to explain weight changes. If the numbers don't add up, look for sources of error in your reporting.

I've often reviewed patients' food journals that indicate they eat less than 1,200 calories per day, yet aren't losing weight. Sometimes patients attribute this lack of weight loss to a slow metabolism, decreased physical activity, or having a Martian-like physiology that defies the laws of thermodynamics. But the true reason is usually based on inaccurate reporting. The most common errors come from waiting too long to record intake, or failing to weigh and measure food. Other patients may be eating a lot of unknown calorie foods. They may frequently stop at a mom-and-pop diner for lunch, and although they do their best to determine portion sizes and calories, they really don't know what's in the food. Lastly, people using electronic apps make mistakes by selecting foods from the database that don't match what they actually consumed.

Consider the peculiar

Spray margarine is a great way to get the flavor of butter without the calories. The primary ingredients are water and oil. If you look at the food label it indicates "0" calories. In fact, it does have calories because it contains oil. But the serving size is "one spray" and rounding the calories of one spray to the nearest digit allows the manufacturer to indicate it has no calories. I've never seen anyone stop after one squirt, but nevertheless, it's a lower-calorie alternative to other added fats.

Tammy, who liked the taste of butter but didn't want the consequences of calories, was an avid food label reader and decided to use spray margarine. In her eyes this was a "free food" because the label clearly read it had zero calories. Since it was calorie-free, she didn't bother putting it in her food journal. Due to great investigative work by one of our registered dietitians, we were able to solve the mystery of why Tammy was gaining weight; she consumed up to two *bottles* of spray margarine every day. She would take off the spray top and pour it on almost everything she ate. This gross-me-out use of spray margarine obviously contributed to her unexplained weight gain.

Another client asked me if she needed to include sugar-free gum in her food journal. My first response was "no." Sugar-free gum only has five calories per stick and the act of chewing gum actually burns a few calories and may prevent someone from mindlessly eating snacks. To me, the calories in the gum were a wash. But as we continued to talk, I began to understand she *really* liked gum. In fact, she was compulsive about chewing it. She was an ex-smoker who used gum to deal with anxiety. She would chew a piece of gum just long enough to get the sweet taste from it, and then she would spit it out and get another piece. She was going through five or six of the 10-piece packs per day. She consumed enough sugar-free gum every day to equal the calories in two regular sodas. Although her breath was always great, she wasn't adequately handling the stress of work. She had a good sense of humor about her gum issue but realized this compulsive chewing was contributing to the problem with her weight. We worked together to help her manage stress in better ways.

Remember the spirit of the food journal

The goal of keeping a food journal is to become more aware of your relationship with food, which will help you establish healthy eating habits that lead to weight loss or maintaining a healthier weight. Most people, even those who are successful, don't use the journal every day for the rest of their lives. However, self-monitoring your diet regularly in the early stages of weight loss is extremely important in order to learn more about your eating patterns and educate yourself on where, when, and under what psychological or environmental circumstances you consume extra calories.

Over time you may decide to only record your food during the times you struggle most, such as evenings or weekends. You may eventually stop recording everything you eat and simply have a daily checklist. Others have successfully used food journaling in tandem with self-weighing, only recording their foods when weight begins to climb.

What About Stepping on the Scales?

People have various opinions on weighing and I've heard a lot of arguments for and against it from patients and professionals. When people can't agree about a topic, turning to science is helpful. After all, my gut instinct tells me the earth is flat. Fortunately, researchers have examined the relationship between weight loss maintenance and self-weighing. The overall conclusion is that self-weighing is associated with weight management success and isn't likely to cause psychological problems.

It's true that obsessive weighing can be a sign, but not usually the cause, of certain eating disorders. People with bulimia nervosa and anorexia nervosa sometimes weigh many times per day—after they eat or go to the bathroom, before and after exercise, before bed, immediately after waking, and after drinking fluids. This type of behavior is obviously a symptom of psychological distress and only gets in the way of recovery.

But for most of us, regular weighing can be a helpful way to monitor progress with eating and physical activity. This is especially important for those who don't keep a food journal.

Self-monitoring your diet provides the highest level of awareness related to your weight. You can record the actual calories you consume and compare that to the approximate calories you need. Weighing, by comparison, gives outcome feedback. Although you may not know precisely how many calories you consume every day, you can see the overall balance by looking at changes in your weight over time.

> *Weighing yourself gives outcome feedback; you can see the overall balance of your weight management by looking at weight changes over time.*

Here's one way to look at food journals: We have a minivan, and yes, I look really cool when my wife lets me drive it. The minivan has a fuel economy gauge that shows our average mileage per gallon and how much farther we can drive until we run out of gas. Similarly, a food journal can reveal how I'm using fuel and how many calories I have left for the day.

By comparison, self-weighing is more like my bare-bones, standard shift Dodge. It has nothing fancy—no power windows or locks and definitely not one of the cool gauges that gives me real-time information about fuel economy. I should mention that it *does* have a radio and cup holders. I can still figure my fuel efficiency after I fill up my tank, observe the change in my odometer, and apply some 6th grade math. Compared to my wife's minivan, which gives immediate feedback, figuring the mileage in my Dodge is like weighing; I get snapshots of how I'm doing between fill-ups. Similar to weighing, I can't isolate the real-time impact of a specific behavior, such as fast starts while driving through town or using cruise control. (That is, if I *had* cruise control).

Although being aware of fuel economy can alert you to potential problems associated with your car, it's not the same as body weight. You don't feel disgusted with your car if your miles per gallon drop off in the winter, and you aren't likely to hide fuel efficiency numbers from your spouse. For some people, numbers on the scale evoke negative emotions and this becomes a monumental barrier to self-weighing. I once worked with a client named Mary, who had worked as a flight attendant in her 20s. Like many other airlines at that time, her employer had weight restrictions and the all-women crew would be weighed in front of each other and scorned if they approached the limit.

"I was always one of the bigger girls, although I only weighed 125 pounds," she told me with tears in her eyes. "I wish I weighed that now."

Many years later, Mary still had an emotional reaction when she stepped on the scale, especially if her weight increased. These weren't just numbers, they meant something to her; they quantified her competence and worth. But avoiding the scale was also problematic. Although she suspected her weight was going up because her clothes fit differently and she could see it in the mirror, this feedback was less frequent and more vague than regular weighing. She had difficulty seeing the short-term cause and effect of her behavior, and therefore she continued to gain weight. We discussed how it was *possible* for her to lose weight and keep it off without ever weighing herself again. But that approach would make things much more difficult. After all, the scale can be a helpful tool that provides information related to our health. Like a true friend, the scale won't always give us the feedback we want, yet it can help us change in a positive direction if we pay attention to the data it provides.

Just as a physician wouldn't tell people with poorly controlled diabetes to avoid checking their blood sugar if high readings make them anxious, I strongly feel professionals should help overweight clients learn to use the scale for their benefit. Although there can be exceptions, I usually advise my clients to weigh no more than once per day, but at least once per week. Weighing first thing in the morning after a trip to the bathroom will minimize the fluctuations you see in weight. I also encourage patients to record their weight on paper or electronically, often using an app, so they can see patterns of weight change and associate those patterns with other aspects of their lives. Recording daily weight can help a woman expect to see a few pounds of water weight gain every month near her menstrual cycle. Knowing this happens every month makes these normal fluctuations less distressing. Seeing a daily weight throughout the holidays can help people think ahead about gatherings and parties in order to maintain weight during the season. When stressful work or family events impact our lives, eating can become less structured and mindless. Frequent weighing can pull our attention back to our desired eating and physical activity habits. In upcoming chapters we'll review how to deal with negative thoughts that keep us off the scale and off track.

Tracking Physical Activity

You're busy, but are you physically active? This may be a tough question. Perhaps you have a sedentary, yet high-paced job that leaves you feeling drained at the end of the day. This tired feeling can fool us into thinking we're more physically active than we really are. If you exercise regularly, you probably have a good idea of how much time you spend being active, but how does all of that add up when you consider what you do the other 15 hours of the day when you're awake? A fitness tracking device can help answer these questions. Wearables include wrist worn devices, pedometers that can be attached to a belt, bra or shoe, and activity trackers built into your smartphone.

Of course you can be active without using devices, and having one doesn't guarantee you'll be more dynamic. But paying attention to the numbers does make you more aware of physical activity patterns. Just as a food journal helps you become more mindful of eating, a wearable fitness device such as those made by Fitbit, Jawbone, Misfit, Garmin (and three other companies that have likely emerged since I started writing this sentence) can provide feedback on your physical activity and help you set objective goals.

I was leading a weight management class on the topic of was physical activity. We compared the pros and cons of exercise and I asked the group why people (and especially overweight folks) often avoid exercise. Karen, who had been quiet and seemingly uninterested in the topic up to that point, chimed in.

"It's torture."

I had turned to write some of the responses on the whiteboard and I wasn't sure if I heard her correctly,

"What was that, Karen?"

"It's torture," she said without a smile.

She actually seemed sort of angry. It was as if people had been telling her to exercise for years but they just didn't understand how terrible it felt for her. Karen was a generally pleasant 40-something lady, about 150 pounds overweight.

"Exercise is exhausting, boring, and it hurts my knees," she said.

As she freely expressed her disdain for exercise, I noticed a bright pink fitness device on her wrist.

"Karen, I notice you have a Fitbit," I said. "Do you like wearing it?"

"I love my Fitbit. It tells me how many steps I've accumulated and I try to reach at least 5,000 per day. I know you're supposed to get 10,000 steps per day but I really can't do that yet. Reaching 5,000 is really an improvement for me. I started taking the stairs down at work and I look for ways to walk around more at home in the evenings. Sometimes if I'm getting close to my step goal, I'll walk my little dog for five or ten minutes in the evening. This thing even tells me how much I move in my sleep."

After hearing her say exercise was torture, I didn't expect her to sing the praises of a wearable fitness device. After a bit more interaction, it became clear that Karen viewed "exercise" as long bouts of intense physical activity at a gym. This didn't appeal to her. On the other hand, she enjoyed accumulating physical activity throughout the day with feedback from her Fitbit. Would it be wonderful if Karen had a change of heart and began a structured exercise program? Sure. But tracking her fitness made her more aware of physical activity and she was setting progressive goals in the right direction.

If you aren't into gadgets or don't want to shell out the money for one, simple fitness tracking techniques can be helpful. Setting a goal to exercise 20 minutes during 20 out of 30 days a month can easily be tracked on a calendar. Each "X" is one step closer to your goal. Other people have set distance goals, planning to walk the equivalent of 500 miles in a year. Every day they mark down their mileage, knowing that ten miles per week keeps them on target. Some of our patients have even placed thumbtacks on a map to show how far they've gone toward their planned destination.

"Going with the flow" of society's eating and exercise habits probably won't lead to long-term weight loss. Instead, we must be intentional about changing our habits. One of the first steps in this process is to pay closer attention to eating and physical activity. When we track our weight, diet, and movement, we heighten our awareness so that progress is clear. This self-monitoring forces us to decide between the short-term pleasures of food and inactivity, and the long-term benefits of restraint and self-discipline—the topic of our next chapter.

Chapter 5

Redefining Pleasure

STEPPING ON THE scale, noting food intake in a journal, and wearing a fitness tracker can remind us of goals and provide feedback on progress. These self-monitoring tools make us aware—they make the facts unavoidable. But simply becoming more aware of our behavior may not be enough to permanently improve our relationship with food and physical activity.

It may sound a bit odd to say we have a relationship with food, but most of us do. We're connected to it in meaningful ways. Granted, some people primarily view food as fuel to keep the body going while they focus on other things. This can be true for those who are intensely focused on health and physical performance. For them, eating is like going to the gas station to fill the tank. I don't know anyone who has a relationship with food exactly like this, but some athletes are the closest match. For focused, dedicated athletes, food can be part of a training regimen where the pleasure of eating is less important than their competition goals.

> *Most of us have a complex link to food. We eat for a variety of reasons, beyond hunger or providing the highest quality fuel for our bodies.*

Most of us have a more complex link to food. We eat for a variety of reasons beyond hunger or providing the highest quality fuel for our bodies. For a moment, put aside thoughts of eating to appease hunger and provide energy. What else determines whether or not you eat something? What factors lead you to stop eating once you've started? You may find the next several chapters most helpful if you make an actual list of what influences your food choices and portions.

If we reviewed your list, we could probably place most of your reasons into one of three general categories: pleasure, coping, and the environment. As we explore these three categories in the upcoming chapters, remember they can be combined and multifaceted. Eating when you aren't hungry can have multiple triggers. For now, let's focus on our internal drives to eat and begin to redefine the pleasure of eating.

Pleasure

Cindy was a relatively quiet member of the weekly weight loss group I led. The mother of two small boys, she held a professional position at a local accounting firm. Her stylish clothing helped conceal the extra 30 pounds she was never able to lose after her youngest son, now four years old, was born. She wore tasteful makeup to accentuate her short brown hair and light complexion.

Between the group meetings, I would meet alone with each client to review progress and talk about the changes each patient hoped to make. During this private time people could share things they didn't want to discuss with the group. Cindy arrived on time to one of our individual appointments, wearing an attractive, calf-length blue dress with a white floral pattern. After a brief discussion of how she thought the group meetings were going, she began to reveal why she hadn't lost weight since beginning the program: Chocolate. Lots of chocolate.

"I like the good stuff," she exclaimed as she began describing her square little friends. "They aren't like the typical chocolates you can pick up at any grocery store." She went on to explain how the chocolates tantalized her as she removed them from the appealing European wrappers, unleashing a provocative, sweet scent before she took a bite.

"Have you ever had this type of chocolate?" she asked.

I admitted I had not. In fact, I felt a little uncultured because I'd never heard of it. I thought Hershey Kisses looked fancy in their foil wrappers. Cindy was about to show me that not all chocolates are created equal. In fact, she described consuming chocolate in a poetic fashion, full of imagery and passionate voice inflection. By the time she finished portraying the smooth shiny texture, the perfect balance between sweet and bitter flavor, the slowly melting, creamy mouthfeel, and the notes of flavor that lingered in her mouth after each piece, I was ready to get on a plane to Belgium, or wherever this stuff was made.

From my outsider point of view, Cindy's chocolate eating was an experience filled with anticipation and naughtiness. This was her private, Calgon-take-me-away, Herbal-Essence-shampoo moment. Cindy's problem wasn't that she loved chocolate; it was the fact that chocolate became a primary source of pleasure in her life—and not once in a while. It happened every day. One piece led to multiple pieces and the calories added up.

Not everyone has a single food they use, or abuse, in this way. Other clients have a time of day—usually evening or mid-afternoon, when different foods provide pleasure and relaxation from the day's stressful experiences. Some people combine two pleasurable activities to heighten the satisfaction of the experience, such as eating while watching TV, reading, or watching sports.

Some of us eat to neutralize something unpleasant or boring. A college student may devour a bag of chips while studying for a chemistry exam; your boss may bring doughnuts into work during a high-volume work season; or a church may entice you to join a Bible study group by offering food. I was surprised when a church I attended for a short time started a group named "Gab and Gorge." No joke! I opted out and wondered if they would start a "Smoke and Serve" or "Drink and Disciple" group.

Finding pleasure in food is a good thing. If we didn't enjoy our food, how would we eat enough to survive? Unpleasant hunger feelings and the reward of eating motivated our ancestors to hunt, gather, and preserve food. But the advent of refrigeration, high-speed transportation and mass processing led to easy-access food in extremely palatable forms. Today, we need little motivation or effort to obtain food. We can order groceries online or have a pizza delivered by sending a text. This is a far cry from what my great grandmother did to prepare a meal. If we wanted fried chicken, she would walk out the back door, choose the unlucky bird, and then proceed to wring its neck, pluck the feathers, and remove its innards.

> *For many of us, eating has progressed from a pleasurable necessity to a leisure-time activity.*

In modern society our inherent drive to eat can become distorted. Because food is pleasurable and easy to get, we must be aware of what, and how much, we consume in order to avoid weight gain. For many of us, eating has progressed from a pleasurable necessity to a leisure-time activity. It's easy to fall into the trap of using food as entertainment. Food, unlike other things people use for pleasure, is legal, readily available, inexpensive, and socially acceptable. In addition, the reward from eating something savory is almost instantaneous as it makes contact with the taste buds on our tongues. In psychological terms, that instant pleasure is a primary reinforcer. We don't have to learn about its value, because we experience the innate, biological benefit. Offer a 3-year old a choice between candy or a twenty-dollar bill and you'll see what I mean.

> *Many overweight people experience hunger and fullness in a different way than people who are normal weight.*

To further complicate things, many overweight people experience hunger and fullness in a different way than people who are normal weight. Some people crave food the same way a compulsive gambler yearns for the rush of a big win. Losing weight can make things even more difficult from a physiological standpoint. Our body reacts to weight loss in a manner that influences us to quickly regain those pounds. Metabolism drops and neurochemicals that impact appetite respond in ways that favor weight regain. In many ways, your body tells the brain, "Hey, we're starving!" The brain defends your weight, even if you weigh too much. If only our brains had a built-in scale that promoted weight loss and maintaining a healthy weight, but that doesn't appear to be the case. Here's part of how the system works:

The body's chemical response to weight loss

With weight loss, a hunger hormone called ghrelin (produced in the stomach) begins to increase. Receptors in the brain take notice and create a propensity for regaining weight.

Leptin is a protein produced by fat cells. It tells the brain you've eaten enough. Leptin decreases with weight loss and makes keeping weight off a challenge. Ghrelin and leptin are two of many hormones and neurochemicals that make losing and maintaining weight loss so difficult. The body's tendency to fight weight loss is much more complicated than just leptin, ghrelin, and metabolic changes; but we know the brain, primarily the hypothalamus, is the conductor of the eat-more orchestra.

Other parts of the brain, especially a region called the nucleus accumbens, are involved with different pleasures, including pleasure from food.

Researchers refer to the desire for pleasurable foods in the absence of an energy (calorie) deficit as "hedonic hunger." Like the urges of a drug addict, hedonic hunger can be intense. Certain foods have a high "hedonic rating" and some people are more susceptible than others to this type of eating.

How to make smart decisions

Knowing that parts of the brain keep nudging us to gain weight is helpful, but that isn't the end of the story. Fortunately, the human brain and our behavior go beyond urges and pleasure seeking. Just as a visually impaired person can fine tune other senses, a person whose brain tends to promote obesity can develop other neural pathways that help with weight management. Regions of the brain such as the prefrontal cortex help us make smart decisions and resist temptation that may harm us or others.

So how do we combat the internal drive to overeat, which is often stronger for people who struggle with obesity than for people of normal weight? Many clients tell me they just have to stop using food for pleasure—they need to be disciplined. They white-knuckle it and lose weight. But over time, *all work and no play makes Jack a dull boy*. People who've lost weight sometimes feel over-restrained, rigid, and pleasure deprived. This is a recipe for relapse into old patterns of eating. In order to avoid these feelings and the weight regain that often results, we must find alternative pleasures in our life. To explore this further, I'd like you to make a list of things you find pleasurable.

Some of your items, such as travel or hobbies you do away from home, may require appointments, planning, and money. Put them on your list. But because food is so readily available, we need to find healthy substitutes that are also easy to do, convenient, and low-cost. If it's late in the evening and ice cream starts calling your name, you can't exactly get on a cruise to the Caribbean. You need a simpler alternative. Below are 20 simple activities patients have used as a substitute for pleasure eating. Obviously we want to refine the list by including only items that are incompatible with eating and aren't unhealthy in other ways (such as smoking). If you tend to mindlessly consume food while using the computer, or drink a margarita while getting a foot rub, you may want to take those off your list. For items not immediately within reach, thinking about them or taking action to prepare for them can be a great substitute for eating. For instance, planning for a vacation may be a great way to distract yourself from a late-night cookie craving.

I encourage you to continuously add new activities to your list. When you have an urge to eat because you're bored, do something from your list instead. When you're wandering the kitchen looking for "something that tastes good" but you're not hungry, check your list. With time, you'll likely develop regular hobbies and routines that keep you busy and fulfilled—a role food used to play. These are sample activities other people have noted:

Reading	Listening to music	Playing with kids/grandkids	Taking a walk
Playing with dog	Crocheting	Scrapbooking	Playing games
Getting online	Organizing	Taking a bath	Lighting a candle
Planning a trip	Napping	Hanging out with friends	Writing
Talking to others	Riding bikes	Doing puzzles	Getting a massage

What is pleasure?

What if you decided to redefine *pleasure*? Changing your ideas about what makes you feel good can be an excellent strategy to help you stop eating for pleasure. The flavor, texture, and presentation of food are only small parts of the "pleasure package" we get from eating. Imagine yourself eating a scrumptious dish with your best friend at your favorite restaurant. This is an "I could eat this every day for the rest of my life" dinner. You've ordered everything you love from the menu, including appetizers and high-calorie drinks, and have plans for an amazing dessert. After the third bite of this elegant meal you close your eyes, move your head from side to side. "Mmmm. Perfection."

But when you open your eyes, the food paradise comes to a screeching halt. Out of your peripheral vision you notice something scampering across the floor near your feet. "Ew, it's a cockroach!" you whisper forcefully to your friend as you lift your feet off the floor. With your knees held high, you attract the attention of other diners. When you make eye contact with one of them, you see another unwelcome guest— the man at the next table has a cockroach crawling up the sleeve of his shirt. He has no clue and continues eating and glancing over *at you* with curiosity. You quickly look away, trying to spot a server you can alert. Now you see cockroaches on the wall. In less than five seconds, which seems more like five minutes, you locate your server. Your stomach churns as you make another unbelievable observation: A cockroach on her nametag? Disgusting!

Just for kicks, imagine you, the man at the other table, and the server all notice the problem and either smash the little critters and dispose of them—or trap them in a glass and let them loose outside if that makes you feel better. The roaches on the walls crawl through the small spaces in the crown molding. No more roaches in sight. Everything appears perfectly normal now. You can get back to your wonderful meal, right? Uh, no. I'm just guessing you may want to leave. Do you want a to-go container? Not a chance. Will you come back next week? I doubt it. How about getting that same dish at another restaurant? Probably not.

This is a silly example I hope you'll never experience. But let's think about why you're suddenly not interested in a dish that seemed like the greatest food ever. The flavor hasn't changed, but your thinking moved from one end of the spectrum to another. Now you're considering insect droppings in your food and the prospects of getting sick. Even the dinner rolls look suspicious, though their flavor hasn't changed.

> *The eating experience changes forever when we begin thinking about our food as more than flavor.*

The eating experience changes forever when we begin thinking about our food as more than flavor; when we consider how it nourishes our bodies, what it's doing for us (or to us), where it came from, and how we're going to feel after eating.If you blindfold me and asked me to rate the amount of pleasure I experience when eating a McDonald's french fry compared to a carrot stick, the french fry always wins. But if you tell me I'm about to eat a carrot grown in your backyard that you picked, rinsed, and cut up just for me; that its nutrients will help with eyesight, immunity, and muscle contraction; and you remind me to notice the earthy, refreshing flavor as I bite into it—my pleasure meter rises quite a bit from the carrot.

By comparison, you might remind me the tasty french fry contains hydrogenated oil, sodium acid pyrophosphate, tertiary butylhydroquinone, and dimethylpolysiloxane. The fry may contribute to weight gain, which could lead to diabetes or high blood pressure that requires medication with side effects like tiredness or sexual dysfunction. Suddenly I no longer experience as much pleasure from the french fry.

My former client Rachel has an advanced degree in communications and a wonderful ability to make friends, work a crowd, and entertain at home. She could easily become your lifetime friend after sitting next to her on a flight or sharing a cab. But her lifestyle of work-related travel, frequent dining out, and inactivity contributed to a long-term battle with her weight. Despite her professional success and many friends, Rachel's weight was the thing she hated most about herself. Her goal, like many other driven, results-oriented people, was to change her life in a way she could sustain.

Changing her approach to dining out was one thing she worked on during our time together. Knowing excess calories often come from the appetizers, sides, or condiments, she made her own rule not to eat french fries at meals. Her favorite line when speaking to her server was, "I'm allergic to french fries. Can I get something else?"

Occasionally a server would ask, "Really, you're allergic to french fries. What happens if you eat them?"

"Oh, it's terrible," Rachel would say. "I break out in fat, all over my body!"

This type of thinking can shed a different light on food and the pleasure we derive from it. The broccoli Rachel ordered as her side was pleasurable, not only because it tasted good, but also because it reminded her of all the things she could do when she was healthy. That broccoli prevented her "allergic reaction."

Food is supposed to be pleasurable, but its primary purpose is to nourish us. As we learn to fuel our bodies for meaningful and fulfilling activities, our relationship with food changes. Expanding pleasure, rather than eliminating it from our lives, is one way to make weight loss sustainable. Although finding alternative pleasures is important, it may not be enough to keep us on track when life is at its hardest. In the next chapter, we'll explore ways to sustain health when emotions run high.

Chapter 6

Letting Go of Emotional Eating

PEOPLE COMMONLY USE food to deal with stress. After all, food is an enjoyable distraction and easy to find. When you feel stressed at work, a vending-machine candy bar may only be steps from your office. At home, our well-stocked pantries and refrigerators make emotional eating an easy way to cope. And once in the kitchen, what foods call to us? It certainly isn't lettuce or carrots. Most likely we hear a siren song from ice cream, chips and salsa, cake, or some other high-calorie food.

One TV commercial shows a sniffling, downtrodden young woman paying for items at a convenience store. She places ice cream, potato chips, and a box of tissues on the counter. The elderly cashier empathetically says, "Oh, honey, he broke up with you again?" Viewers understand this because emotional eating is so common. This young woman is using food to deal with sadness, abandonment, and anger.

In my weight management groups and individual sessions with people trying to lose weight, I frequently ask, "What influences you to eat when you aren't hungry?"

Many people respond by saying, "I'm an emotional eater." Even among those who deny emotional eating, we often discover patterns of weight gain during stressful times and life transitions that suggest otherwise. And it's not just negative stress – positive stress also can influence eating and physical activity. Exciting life transitions, sometimes referred to as eustress, can impact our behavior. These stressors may include the birth of a child, a job promotion, a new house, or a new relationship. We might gain weight because we party and stop exercising at college, take on the unhealthy habits of a spouse during our first year of marriage, use food as entertainment when we travel, or celebrate anything and everything with cake. Over time, eating during periods of eustress or distress becomes a pattern that seems normal. We eat without much awareness of the circumstances and emotions that contribute to our food choices.

Redefining pleasure, the topic of the last chapter, can help us eat healthy during times of celebration and still enjoy life. Monitoring weight, physical activity, and diet (Chapter 4) can keep us from veering off track during exciting times. But for many people, persistent distress is more connected to unhealthy weight than positive stress. With or without awareness, stressed-out employees, moms and dads, college students, and even children self-medicate with food. The remainder of this chapter will primarily focus on maintaining healthy behavior when we experience negative emotions.

I don't want to turn you into an unemotional robot when it comes to eating. I do want to help you become intentional about how you react to stress. Being deliberate and aware of our reactions is often a challenge, because the interaction between emotions and eating is complex. Fortunately, we can begin making positive changes without understanding every detail of why we eat.

To simplify, let's accept that emotions impact everyone's eating habits to a certain degree. Your unique patterns may be so ingrained that you barely notice them. To better understand your patterns, it may help to answer the following questions:

- How often do you emotionally eat?
- When do you tend to do this (evenings, weekends, or when your mother-in-law visits)?

- How much food (and what) do you usually eat?
- At the time, do you realize you're eating because of your emotional state or is it more like a mindless grazing pattern?
- Do you lose your appetite when you're stressed but then end up overeating when you finally relax?
- Do you intentionally plan emotional eating (making sure you'll be alone or have your preferred foods)?
- Do you eat until you're uncomfortably full and/or feel out of control?

As the questions above illustrate, people have different patterns of emotional eating. You may be a grazer—tasting food as you hurriedly prepare dinner or inching your way through a sleeve of crackers while helping a reluctant child complete his homework. Maybe you tend to not eat when you're stressed, but overcompensate later when the pressures of life subside. Or you may be a frequent binge eater, consuming food until you're uncomfortably full, feeling out of control and only eating in private, and feeling embarrassed and guilty when you finish. If the last sentence describes you, consider seeking professional help. A therapist skilled in eating disorders can help you better understand your behavior and guide you to incorporate the suggestions included in this chapter.

Does Emotional Eating Help?

Do we feel better after eating to deal with negative emotions? To a certain degree the food must help, because we keep doing it. But what's the function of food in this scenario? In most cases eating creates a pleasurable distraction from our emotional discomfort. Unfortunately, the worry or anger is sure to return after we're stuffed with food. Yet, many people condition themselves to eat when they're stressed by doing it over and over—consuming something pleasurable in a soothing environment to momentarily cover their uncomfortable feelings.

Jeff inherited his grandmother's home after she died. In a sad set of circumstances, she had raised him after he was removed from his biological mother's house. Grandma loved him dearly and expressed this in one of the only ways she knew how—with food. Jeff especially loved her homemade noodles served over mashed potatoes made with sour cream and butter. As a result of a genetic predisposition, the trauma of his childhood, and day-to-day eating habits at his grandmother's home, Jeff became morbidly obese. His large size created so much knee and back pain he was forced to leave his job and go on disability, for which he receives a modest disability check each month. How does Jeff deal with his chronic pain, plus depression over not having a job or an intimate relationship? He cooks in the same kitchen as his grandmother, and frequently makes noodles and mashed potatoes—his comfort food. Eating will temporarily help Jeff forget his situation and comfort him with memories of his grandmother. But like most emotional eating, it only makes his situation worse in the long run. His chronic pain will continue to worsen and he won't be able to work if he continues using food to cope with his circumstances.

Solving Problems versus Enduring Them

Some of you may be like Tina. She had lost about 25 pounds and was at the upper end of a healthy weight range. Like many people in her situation, she wanted to lose 15 more pounds, but she looked and felt healthy. Tina is extremely organized and approaches life with to-do lists, specific goals, and step-by-step action plans to achieve them. She is aware of her struggles with excess calories, which mainly sneak in from sweets or too much weekend alcohol.

After seeing Tina for over two years, the two of us became remarkably good at solving problems related to her eating issues. She made food plans for weekend excursions, holidays, and dining out. At social gatherings she worked hard to stick to her one to two drink maximum. She maintained a workout routine by attending group fitness classes. When a problem arose, she took a systematic approach and solved it.

But life threw Tina an unhittable curveball when her husband was diagnosed with late-stage cancer. Suddenly she faced a problem she couldn't solve. All her planning and strategies couldn't make this go away. She was not in control. As a result, Tina began losing focus and started regaining weight. The energy she usually put into mindful eating, planning for high-risk situations, and practicing restraint was now being used in an attempt to solve an unsolvable problem—cancer. Trying to solve unsolvable problems looks a lot like worry and can lead to feeling anxious and depressed.

Like Tina, we all encounter situations we can't fix; from bad weather or the performance of a sports team, to serious issues such as children with drug abuse problems, an alcoholic spouse, illness, chronic pain, or fallout from a childhood riddled with sexual, physical, or emotional abuse.

Tina was skilled at problem-focused coping—changing or eliminating the source of stress and putting problem-solving plans into action. But she wasn't very skilled at emotion-focused coping, a skill we all need when a problem can't be fixed. When we attempt to change our emotional reactions to stressful events, we're using emotion-based coping—which can be healthy or unhealthy. Soothing or distracting ourselves with food is an unhealthy way to do this. At this point in her life, Tina needed to maintain her psychological wellbeing by coping with something she couldn't change. Realizing she couldn't alter her husband's cancer diagnosis, Tina once again started using food to regulate her mood and calm her nerves.

With a lot of work, Tina began to accept what she couldn't change. By learning to use a variety of strategies to avoid emotional eating when she felt frustrated or anxious, she was able to stop regaining weight after only a few pounds. She realized that emotional eating is a temporary fix with an undesirable side effect—possible weight gain.

> *Emotion-based coping can be healthy or unhealthy. Our reactions can harm us in the long run, or they can make us stronger.*

Coping with Emotions in a Healthy Manner

"Food is my drug of choice."

I often hear that phrase while working with people who struggle to lose weight. Using food to cope with problems usually leads to later feelings of disappointment, anxiety, and even self-loathing. The cycle of "feel stressed, overeat, feel bad, overeat again" may continue for years and even become a way of life. The only way to break this cycle is by finding other, more productive, less harmful, ways to deal with emotional issues. Later I'll discuss how modifying thoughts and beliefs can prevent us from feeling overwhelmed. But for now, let's assume you're already feeling pressured, threatened, sad, angry, anxious, or browbeaten. How can you cope?

First, consider the list of healthy, pleasurable activities you created in the previous chapter. Using a delightful distraction like reading, crocheting, or working on a car remodel can provide temporary relief similar to the comfort and distraction you get from food. Adding to your list of alternative activities may help you with eating issues. Consider new hobbies you'll enjoy—things you've always wanted to try. Don't let your weight stand in the way of trying something new.

These activities promote relaxation and offer temporary relief. But some situations, especially ongoing sources of discontent, are best handled when we *process the stress* rather than distract ourselves from it. Developing coping mechanisms beyond food is the best way to find peace in spite of undesirable feelings and events. Distractions only scratch the surface of our discontent, like applying a small Band-Aid to a deep cut. Effective emotion-focused coping often requires deeper processing of what's happening. That includes learning to tell which problems we can solve, versus problems we need to live with for a while. For example, the illness of Tina's husband wasn't something she could change. She could best handle her worry by calming herself and finding peace within a different perspective. Similarly, Jeff had issues from childhood that problem solving could help but wouldn't immediately or completely resolve.

I admit, coping strategies that aren't distractions may not be enjoyable in themselves, because you're facing problems instead of avoiding emotional pain. Creating a relaxed environment for coping activities will help you glean as much immediate contentment from them as possible.

Journaling

Journaling has become a wildly popular activity in our culture. Your journal can be a friend who always listens and never says hurtful things. Writing in those pages can help you explore what lies behind feelings such as fear, anger, and pain. Getting specific about things that bother you can help erase superficial worry and uncover more deep-seated issues. With complete privacy, you can explore the past, let go of it, and begin planning for the future. No one has to see your irrational tirades or words that could hurt others. You can edit, keep those pages, or throw them away. Later you might re-read the journal and notice your own faulty reasoning.

But if a journal is only a punching bag of sorts where you vent anger, frustration, and pain, it may not live up to its potential for helping you through stressful times. The goal of journaling is to find meaning, clarity, and eventually peace. Ending some entries by completing statements such as:

"something helpful I'm learning is . . ."

"this probably happened because . . ."

"I want to use this experience to . . ."

"I can start letting go of this because . . ."

"I will be kind to myself because . . ."

. . .can make journaling more therapeutic. You might also finish a painful entry by redirecting your thoughts to the most meaningful parts of your life—things that bring joy, things you're proud of, and things you look forward to doing.

In addition to your regular journal, keeping a special gratitude journal can direct your thoughts away from negativity and toward the things you're most thankful for. Writing in detail about people who've blessed our lives, possessions we're grateful for, and experiences that have helped us grow can be uplifting and get us through tough times.

Talking to others

As an alternative to emotional eating, relying on close friends or family members who are good listeners and rational responders can help you deal with stress. Sometimes a quick, supportive phone call or text message can be enough to pull you through a difficult moment. However, keep in mind that friendship and family relationships are two-way streets. If you feel your conversations are burdening others, seek professional help. Therapists not only listen, but can guide you to develop coping skills and manage life in a healthier manner.

Religious-based coping

Although religious practices and beliefs vary a great deal, most people worldwide believe in God or a higher power. The concept of an all-knowing, ever present, loving God is beyond our ability to fully grasp. This can be frustrating and confusing at times, yet accepting this belief can give us a great sense of peace.

When I was a child my family often took summer trips to the beach, which was a 14-hour drive when we were "driving straight through" and "making good time." Sometimes we left home at 2:00 or 3:00 a.m. so we could check into our hotel in the afternoon. On the way back home we usually left around noon and arrived home a few hours before sunrise. Although my dad drove for many hours through mountains, heavy thunderstorms, and congested traffic, I never worried about safely arriving. I knew Dad would get us there. With no worries at all, I fell asleep alongside my brother and sister—who, by the way, always took more than her fair share of the large back seat in our Chrysler New Yorker. If you believe in an all-powerful God who has your best interests in mind, then you can relate to the peacefulness I felt while riding in our car.

An old saying tells us, "God can move mountains, but bring your shovel." This is true most of the time. However, sometimes we simply need to wait and trust that, although life brings unexpected and painful turns, we will be okay in the end, even if the pathway is a journey we wouldn't have chosen. In order to wait more effectively, we can pray, meditate, read faith-based literature, attend services, and socialize with others who remind us to embrace the idea that in the end something helpful will result from our difficult situation.

Exercise

Physical activity can relieve anxiety as well as treat and prevent depression. Studies even suggest regular physical activity compares in effectiveness to medications used to treat some mood disorders.

Combining activity with something else you find enjoyable can also be an effective coping strategy. Walking or working out with a friend, taking a group fitness class, walking your dog, or finding a scenic place to ride a bike or walk can enhance your experience and help you deal with life difficulties. On the other hand, don't underestimate the benefits found in the solitude of exercise. Even walking on a treadmill in a dark basement can be a time of reflection that leaves you more energized and able to think and solve problems more effectively.

Breathing

When we're upset about something, focusing on our breathing is the simplest thing we can do to calm ourselves. Feeling stressed causes us take shallow, rapid breaths as the body's fight-or-flight response kicks in. You'll also notice a tendency to clench your jaw, furrow your brow, and tense your shoulders. This is the body's automatic response to a threat, whether the threat is physical or emotional. When you're facing an emotional situation, do you really need to run or fight? Instead, you probably want to relax and calm down. Instead of using food to feel better, try focusing on a simple technique you can do anywhere: Deep breathing. This diaphragmatic/belly breathing can slow the heart rate, decrease blood pressure, and calm your nerves. Here's how to do it: Let your abdomen expand as you deeply inhale. Take the air in through your nose and release it slowly through pursed lips, while visualizing your muscles relaxing. You might also focus on accepting healing light as you inhale and releasing tension with each exhale. For better results, combine this with soothing music, yoga, or other relaxation activities.

> *Instead of using food to feel better, try focusing on a simple technique you can do anywhere: Deep breathing*

Helping Others

When you're dealing with issues that won't go away overnight, consider helping other people with their problems. This may sound counter-intuitive, but it works. No matter what our circumstance, we can usually find others who are worse off. Feeding the homeless, volunteering at a women's shelter, or assisting at a school, church, or hospital can take you away from your own issues and give you a sense of purpose. Plus, you'll meet new people and possibly make friends, while making the world a better place.

Although helping others won't erase your problems, it may give you a different perspective. When I help transport someone in a wheelchair it's easier for me to accept the moderate amount of pain in my arthritic joints. When I help families of children with cognitive or physical limitations, my own children's meltdowns are put into perspective. Providing a backpack with school supplies for a child of an inner-city family reminds me of how fortunate I truly am.

Medication

For some people, taking medication is a helpful strategy for coping with stress and psychological conditions. Although you may want to try other strategies first, medication has a place for treating anxiety, depression, and mental illness. You shouldn't feel ashamed or embarrassed if your doctor prescribes something to help. However, don't forget that medication is never a substitute for healthy coping; rather, it should be used to make healthy coping easier.

Chapter 7

Our Environment

AFTER HAVING TWIN boys, Ted and Linda hoped to become pregnant again. Neither of them hid their desire for a little girl. After five years of trying, they accepted that another child wasn't in the cards for them. Once they reached their 40s, Ted and Linda were enjoying their teenage boys and had long given up on trying to increase the size of their family. Then they received amazing news—Linda was pregnant—and they were having a girl! They named her Emily, a name they picked out ten years earlier.

For the first five years of her life Emily lived in a fast-paced home, often eating on the run and snacking on junk food like her brothers. She accompanied her parents as they traveled out of town to watch the boys play tennis and baseball. During these trips everyone ate fast food and consumed not-so-healthy snacks. Soon after Emily's sixth birthday her brothers moved away to college. Emily and her family no longer traveled to sporting events and their home life became much calmer. In essence, Emily suddenly became an only child.

I met Emily four years after her brothers moved out of the house, when she was ten and the family no longer needed to eat on the run. Although the always-starving teenage boys hadn't lived there for years, Emily and her parents still ate out frequently and kept the same types of food in the pantry. As a result, Emily had become quite overweight.

Her concerned parents and pediatrician enrolled Emily

in our children's weight management program. Although Emily's mom came to the initial consultation, her work schedule and frequent travel made it difficult for her to attend regular sessions. Since her father Ted did the shopping, meal planning, and cooking as a stay-at-home dad, our staff worked with him in our efforts to help Emily lose weight We soon realized Dad's habits and perspective were a big part of Emily's struggle with her weight. For instance, he regularly purchased large bags of tortilla chips, mainly for his personal late-night snacking. Because *Dad* wanted to keep snack foods in the house for himself, the conversation turned to *Emily's* motivation and self-discipline. Emily respectfully listened to her father and tried to explain she wanted to do well in the program. After her father continued suggesting she could avoid the chips or only have a small serving for her after-school snack, she uncharacteristically snapped at him, "Dad, I have willpower, but I also have arms!"

We can all relate to Emily's sentiment. The environment in which we live can make or break weight loss efforts. While Emily's father wanted her to practice restraint and use willpower, Emily knew the environment was more than she could handle. Focusing on a 10-year-old's willpower seemed a little silly when a more reasonable solution was to modify the food in the pantry. Doing so would also show support for Emily's struggle.

> *The environment in which we live can make or break weight loss efforts*

On the other hand, Emily's father couldn't create a perfect environment, nor can you. At some point we all have to stop blaming the environment and using it to excuse our actions — at least according to a client named Marty.

In a discussion group of 12 people, Marty and I were the only men. One evening, as we discussed the challenges of weight management, ten ladies did a nice job of describing how their home environments, workplaces, and fast-paced lifestyles got in the way. Marty sat quietly for the first half hour, but toward the end of our time he began squirming in his chair. Finally, he sat up straight and sighed loudly to let everyone know he had something on his mind. We all looked at the 40-something chemist who'd gained 50 pounds since beginning work at a pharmaceutical company six years earlier. We already knew his long work hours and the addition of two children to his family created a lifestyle conducive to weight gain. We also knew Marty was irritated with himself for gaining weight and even more frustrated that he had to join a weight management group for help. In a previous session he had told us that obesity treatment seemed "stupid" because the solution was simple—eat less and move more. Now we all eagerly awaited his opinion on why weight management was so difficult. He took another deep breath, probably to swallow the four-letter words on the tip of his tongue.

Marty's frustration showed in his furrowed brow and restless fingers that curled into a fist. "I hear what you're all saying. But never, not once, has someone tackled me, pinned my arms to the floor and shoved food down my throat. Never! No person or situation makes us do anything—we're doing this to ourselves."

Marty had a valid point. Despite our food-centric society, we all have freedom to make choices. Although I've heard more than a few troubling stories from my patients about being forced to eat as children, most adults are entirely free to refuse food, or eat in whatever quantities they want. Although the environment can limit our options or make certain behavior difficult to carry out, it does not *force* us to do anything. If we intentionally pay attention to hunger, fullness, our calorie needs, and the nutritional quality of our food, we can maintain a healthy diet despite the availability and ease of obtaining highly pleasurable, unhealthy foods.

But we live in a fast-paced world where it's difficult to always self-monitor every food decision; to constantly be on alert regarding our calorie budgets and how well we're sticking to them. Instead of being proactive, we easily get distracted and just react to our surroundings. In most industrialized nations the surroundings are obesogenic—teeming with food and conveniences that promote obesity.

> *In most industrialized nations the surroundings are obesogenic—teeming with food and conveniences that promote obesity.*

In the United States, two-thirds of adults are overweight or obese, at least partly because of the environment we created. Consistent with human instincts, we tend to make choices based on what's available, convenient, pleasurable, and socially acceptable. It's no stretch to say that unhealthy foods are easier to find than healthier alternatives—think restaurants, gas stations, vending machines, sporting events, and the check-out lines of grocery stores.

Adding to the problem, modern technology has engineered physical activity out of our lives. Many of us drive to work and then sit at desks most of the day. We drive home, push the garage door opener, and walk a short distance to the mailbox. Exhausted from our busy-but-inactive day, we spend another few hours relaxing in front of the TV. To change the channel, we push a button on the remote control. We even have robotic vacuum cleaners to clean our floors and entertain the cat. We take escalators and moving walkways to get through airports, perhaps to conserve energy for putting our tray tables in the upright position.

Sometimes our environment promotes unhealthy eating and inactivity at the same time. The Indiana State Fair, and most other state fairs, offer excellent examples. In Indianapolis, a long trolley pulled by an enormous John Deere tractor gives free rides around the fairgrounds. This is a helpful service for people with disabilities, but healthy people also jump at the opportunity to save a few steps. The remarkable part of this is that many people go to the fair primarily to sample the food. So a trolley provides transportation to the corn dog hut only to pick you up and take you to another area where you can have an elephant ear, a fried Snickers bar, deep fried macaroni and cheese, or a funnel cake. If you get too hot waiting for the trolley you can purchase a giant cup of lemonade filled with a little fresh squeezed lemon and a fourth cup of sugar. Bottled water is always an option, but it costs almost as much as the lemonade, and besides, it *is* the State Fair.

This all seems normal, even to those of us in the health field. When I attend large obesity or fitness conferences I like to observe the behavior of attendees. People leave a presentation with many good ideas after hearing a talk on the benefits of decreasing sedentary behavior and increasing patients' motivation for physical activity. After they leave the room to go to another part of the conference hall, where they will again sit through a 90-minute symposium, they need to go up or down to another floor. When these attendees reach the escalator with a spacious carpeted set of stairs beside it, almost everyone stops walking and rides the escalator. This shows me how persuasive the environment is, even among people who are highly educated on the benefits of healthy behavior.

Obesity in Our Society—the Macro Environment

The obesity epidemic has attracted wide public attention and federal, state, and local governments are taking steps to stop its growth. Obesity and obesity-related diseases, such as diabetes, cost Medicare and Medicaid over 90 billion dollars each year—expenses that are passed on to taxpayers. These programs are becoming harder to fund because, although modern medicine helps keep us alive, the costs are tremendous. Medication, cardiac procedures, joint replacements, and even bariatric surgery are not cheap. If we don't rein in healthcare spending, the benefits programs may cease to exist in a form that provides adequate service. In addition, the heavier and sicker we become as a society, fewer people are able to work and pay taxes to keep funding the programs. The government realizes our national security may be at stake because obesity is such a problem among young adults that our military struggles to recruit young men and women fit enough to serve.

The government passes laws and funds initiatives to create a better environment for healthy eating and active lifestyles. Labeling laws, legislation to control the food served in schools, soda taxes, building walkable communities, and trail projects have potential to benefit the health of society as a whole. But these laws will always be tempered by our nation's high regard for personal freedom. Because of this, legislation and public programs are not going to drastically change our environment. Potato chips, giant burgers with bacon, and all-you-can-eat restaurants won't become illegal anytime soon. Also, public education campaigns, initiatives, and laws compete with the deep pockets of corporations that want to keep us eating their products or streaming services that keep us parked on the couch binge-watching favorite programs.

Aware of insurance costs, absenteeism, and work performance, some employers offer company-wide wellness programs—usually optional services with a financial incentive of some sort. The well-meaning initiatives from government, schools, and employers have an impact on our *macro*-environment. Over time they can change attitudes and our culture—maybe even create a healthier world for our grandchildren. But those of us who want to lose weight in this decade can't depend on the government or workplace to change our environment. We can begin *now* to change our *micro*-environment and make weight management easier.

> *Those of us who want to lose weight can't depend on the government or workplace to change our environments.*

Handling Weight Loss Ourselves—the Micro-Environment

The micro-environment includes your personal relationship with food, the food in your cabinets, grocery shopping practices, the habits of your closest friends and family members, the hours you work, the time you create for physical activity, and the food that's most convenient during high-stress days.

Even the size of your plates, the frequency with which you eat home-cooked meals at the table with family, and how you serve food—family style or pre-plated, can make a difference. Brian Wansink, a prolific researcher in this area, and the author of *Mindless Eating,* puts it this way: "Most of us don't overeat because we're hungry. We overeat because of family and friends, packages and plates, names and numbers, labels and lights, colors and candles, shapes and smells, distractions and distances, cupboards and containers."

My client Suzanne told me she was working hard to pay attention to her hunger and fullness cues, trying to eat only when she was hungry and stop when she was full. At the same time she had an 1,800 calorie per day goal and knew the importance of eating regular meals on a schedule, especially breakfast. But sometimes these strategies were in conflict. Some days she didn't feel like she needed 1,800 calories and other days she was hungrier and truly wanted to eat more. She wanted to know if she should stick to the calorie goal every day no matter how she felt, or should she listen to her body and deviate a bit from the plan. Would her body deceive her and lead her down the path of overeating again? Many days she wasn't hungry until 10 a.m., but wondered if she should go ahead and eat at 6:30 when she awakened.

These are tough questions. As one of my psychology professors once told me, you can respond to most questions with one of three answers: "Money," "Serotonin," or "It depends." Since Suzanne's questions weren't related to why someone did something that compromised their self-dignity, I ruled out the "money" answer. Since her questions were not directly addressing brain activity, I eliminated "serotonin." That left "it depends" as my fallback answer. Primarily, it depends on Suzanne's environment.

In most cases it makes sense to eat within the first hour or two of the day. "Breaking the fast" with breakfast provides energy for the body and fuels the brain. Our metabolisms probably speed up a bit more after eating early, compared to the same food selections later in the day. Research indicates that most successful weight loss maintainers eat breakfast. But waiting a bit longer for your first meal may be okay, depending on the environment. If you're heading to an office where you hit the ground running and doughnuts are waiting in the breakroom, the sweets are tremendously hard to resist on an empty stomach. You may want to eat before you leave home, even if you aren't that hungry. On the other hand, if you have time to microwave a packet of oatmeal you keep in your desk drawer and you have Greek yogurt stored in your work refrigerator, the environment lends itself to success.

Suzanne and I discussed the importance of following a structured plan *and* listening to her body. Balancing the two is much easier when we set up the environment to make the healthiest options the easiest ones.

For an entertaining read related to how the environment can impact eating, I recommend the aforementioned book, *Mindless Eating*, by Dr. Brian Wansink. Much of Brian's research shows how changing the environment can sort of trick us into eating better or worse. If you want to eat less, use a smaller plate. If you want to feel like you're getting more to drink, use a tall thin glass versus a short, wide one. Realize that the larger the bag of pretzels you have, the more you will eat from it, unless you pre-portion your servings. If you want to eat more fruit for snacks, keep a fruit bowl in a high-traffic area. If you're tired of cooking vegetables your young children won't eat, change their names—the vegetables, not your kids. Cook princess peas for your daughter or have your son wash the Ninja Turtle tomatoes that will go in the salad.

Only you can identify what things in your environment create challenges for sustaining a healthy diet. To pinpoint challenges, try working backward from your food journal. When you're eating well, ask yourself, "What in my environment made this easier to do?" When you make regrettable choices, how did the environment cause challenges? If you could relive that day, week, month, or year, how could you create an environment to make healthy eating more likely?

The same assessment strategies can work for physical activity. By understanding when and where you're most likely to be active, you can begin structuring your life to make this easier. Do you need to change your bedtime and get up 30 minutes earlier for exercise, or can you extend your lunch hour and walk at work? If your evenings consist of taxiing children to soccer practice, band, or choir, is there an opportunity to squeeze in exercise? Instead of sitting in the car waiting for your kids, could you walk outside? If you want to watch baseball practice, can you do so while strolling around the field? As discussed earlier, wearing a fitness monitor can be a simple environmental change that spurs you to more activity.

If you enjoy outdoor exercise, have the right equipment to do it year-round. Get an LED light for your bicycle if you want to ride in the winter evenings when it gets dark early. Having the right exercise clothing makes it easier to be flexible and adaptive for all-season exercise. Is it *really* too cold to walk outside? When I worked in Louisiana, clients would sometimes tell me it was too cold for outdoor activity when it was 55 degrees in January. Being a Midwesterner, I never understood this. What I've come to realize is that: 1). Temperature is what we get used to. 2). Having the right apparel (hats, gloves, boots, etc.) is crucial. 3). Weather is a mindset we can either embrace or use as a convenient excuse.

If you live in Buffalo, you'll need a different plan for winter exercise than if you live in Tucson, where the challenge is more about what to do in the summer months. Nevertheless, creating the right environment is important for both places. A Buffalonian may want to invest in walking boots with spikes and a balaclava and mittens for the winter months. For the less adventurous, a gym membership, a treadmill, and a collection of DVDs, or streamed workout videos for home use might be helpful. Tucson residents benefit from loose fitting, lightweight, and light-colored clothing to exercise in the heat. Whether you live in a cool or hot climate, the most important point is your attitude about environmental engineering. Creating the time and will to exercise is more important than the equipment.

Sometimes our environment seems destined to become like the starship *Axiom* in the movie *WAL-E*. It doesn't seem far-fetched to think we can ride everywhere instead of walking, compete virtually rather than physically, and find cupcakes we can drink from a cup. If you haven't seen the movie WAL-E, you can watch it from your computer. (If you hang out with elementary-aged kids you already know that screens are taking over much of our socialization and entertainment, starting at a young age). But we haven't entirely destroyed our planet and we don't live on a spaceship. Even though the environment works against weight management, you can control many things.

Ironically, learning to manage your weight may require avoiding things that are supposed to make life easier—having others prepare and process your food, riding in elevators, spending hours in front of a screen while snacking, etc. But in the end, isn't it worth the effort to structure an environment that fits your personal need to be healthier—not to live easy, but to make healthy living easier? Each of us can do this in some way, even if we start small. If you have good intentions but your thoughts sometimes get in the way of carrying out these plans, keep reading. The next three chapters are especially for you.

SECTION II

IN PREVIOUS CHAPTERS you read how the pleasure of food, our emotions, and the environment can affect food choices and physical activity. We explored ways to find pleasure without food, cope with life's problems in healthy ways, and modify our environments. In most instances, I suggested an observable action on your part—engaging in healthy hobbies, journaling, and placing a fruit bowl in your kitchen, to name a few. The ultimate goal of these strategies is to promote healthy eating and physical activity that leads to sustainable weight loss. But knowing what to do is different than actually doing it. Just as an experienced craftsman with all the right tools may not be able to complete a project, having weight management knowledge and tools doesn't guarantee we'll use them.

Using our weight management tools has a lot to do with things we cannot see—our thoughts, emotions, and beliefs. Because balancing these three factors is crucial to long-term success in weight management, we need to train our brains to help us keep going when things get tough. Your mindset dictates whether you'll use the strategies we've already discussed, or abandon them and fall back into old behavior patterns. Your beliefs will determine whether you regain weight when a family member gets sick, you have financial stress, or the family pet dies. Your emotions related to a hectic work schedule, your teenage daughter's battle with depression, or the death of a parent will determine whether your health goes into a tailspin or you can maintain a healthy lifestyle despite difficult life circumstances. In the next section we'll explore how thoughts, emotions, and behavior are connected and how you can use them to reach your weight management goals.

Chapter 8

The Link between Thoughts, Emotions, and Behavior

HAVE YOU EVER tried to fake having a good time? Even if it's only for a few hours while shopping for window coverings with your wife or walking through an antique car show with your husband, it's hard to pretend you're having fun when you're thinking about a dozen other things you'd rather be doing. Now think about something more long-term, like a job or marriage. If your head isn't into your work or a relationship, you can't pretend things are wonderful day after day. Your behavior will eventually reveal your discontent.

Weight management is the same. If your thoughts, emotions, and behavior are not in sync you won't be able to fake your way through it by using willpower or ignoring your true feelings year after year—that just won't work. How long will you be able to eat healthy if your thoughts are "this diet is for the birds, I wish I could eat real food" or "I just want to eat the way everybody else eats?" Alcohol treatment circles like Alcoholics Anonymous have a name for this type of disconnect between thoughts and behaviors: a dry drunk. It goes something like this:

For many years Pete couldn't control his drinking. He drank almost every day, much to his wife's chagrin. Occasionally he white knuckled it for a day or two and didn't drink, mainly to show his wife he had no problem and could stop anytime he wanted. He sometimes missed work due to hangovers and oversleeping. Recently things escalated as his boss wrote him up for skipping work and two days later he received his third DWI and went to jail. This time, the judge revoked his driver's license. Needless to say, Pete's wife was not happy, knowing she'd be responsible for driving him to and from work and he wouldn't be able to help take the kids to events. She let him sit in jail for two nights before bailing him out and then gave Pete an ultimatum—quit drinking or the marriage is over.

Not only was Pete getting tough love from his wife, the judge ordered him to alcohol treatment. Getting his license back was possible only if he completed treatment and had clean random urine screens for a prolonged period of time.

How did Pete react to these humiliating events? He got angry. First of all, the cop had no right to pull him over; he was driving fine and just had a broken tail light. From his perspective, no one was in danger. His wife was overreacting as usual—even her own mom agreed she could be too emotional. The judge, well, he was ridiculous. Pete, in his mind, was not like all of the other losers who appeared in court.

Besides the anger, Pete was jealous of his buddies who could seemingly drink without being harassed by a badgering wife, an uptight boss, and overzealous cops looking for a reason to lock people up. But he felt backed into a corner with no other option but to stop drinking so, reluctantly, he did. At the court-mandated AA meeting he sat with arms folded in the back of the room, feeling sorry for himself.

Pete was what we call a *dry* drunk. Dry in the respect that he wasn't drinking, a *drunk* because he still had the thinking patterns of an alcoholic in the throes of denial: a toxic combination of blaming others and rationalization.

What happens with dry drunks? Usually they begin drinking again because their thinking patterns and attitudes have not changed. At some point, a person with Pete's frame of mind glorifies the freedom to drink while ignoring the potential consequences. He takes the first sip and then finishes the drink. Since he's already blown it, he has another. Not only has he already screwed up, but the effects of the alcohol are setting in and that feels good, so he keeps drinking, not for one night, but tomorrow, too. This lapse leads to a complete relapse into old patterns of behavior, all but destroying his confidence to give recovery another attempt.

But there is another possibility. In some cases, a dry drunk will change his thinking patterns and remain sober. Possibly, Pete will begin to notice his mind is clearer, he has more energy, and is getting along with his wife better now that he's sober. He starts to remember why they got together in the first place. He is "present" with his kids and sees what he's been missing all these years. His 9-year-old daughter is so smart and seems to enjoy having grown-up conversations with him. Shooting baskets with his 11-year-old son is much more rewarding than sitting on the couch drinking and watching TV. He hears the news about a drunk driver killing an entire family in an accident and starts to accept that his behavior could have led to the same terrible result. His buddies' lives aren't as great as they once seemed; their marriages and relationships with their kids leave much to be desired. If his positive thoughts about sobriety translate into changed behavior, it's feasible, even likely, that Pete will stay sober.

People cannot easily overcome alcoholism, and Pete's scenario shows that staying sober only happens when we align our thinking with our behavior. Changing both thoughts and behavior takes a lot of courage and hard work.

The same goes for managing weight. Over the years, I've encountered many weight management dry drunks. These folks follow a diet for a while, but what they really want is to eat whatever they want, whenever they want. Following a diet is akin to serving a prison sentence and they feel they're "doing time" for a crime they didn't commit. They tell themselves, or other people tell them, they must follow a certain eating and exercise regimen. Certain foods are off limits and their choices are non-negotiable.

This constant oversight by the food police, whether themselves or others, can lead to sadness, anger, and jealousy. These feelings are often directed at friends or family members who don't have to struggle with weight, despite their poor diets and little exercise. Typical thoughts include:

"I don't know how she stays so thin eating like that—it isn't fair!"

"I can't have any pie because this miserable diet doesn't allow it."

"I have to get on that boring treadmill to burn more calories."

"What's the point in going out to dinner if I can't eat food I like?"

Some of these weight management dry drunks are distressed and saddened by the notion that they can only lose weight by giving up something they love so much—delicious food. Along with these thoughts comes the reality of what will happen if they don't lose weight:

"My doctor said I can't have knee surgery until I lose 50 pounds, and I can't stand this pain."

"I avoid any building that requires walking up stairs and I'm afraid if I fell I couldn't get up—so I have to lose weight."

"I have no choice because I can't bear the thought of someone having to care for me when I get older. It would take two or three people just to lift me."

Like Pete, these people feel backed into corners. They don't really want to change their behavior and often think about the misery associated with dieting, exercise, and paying attention to their weight. They just want to live a "normal" life, but the threat of bad things to come will keep them on track for a while. Yet their heads are not in the game. They are reluctantly meandering away from bad things instead of running toward something they truly desire. Like a child who behaves only to avoid punishment, they are primed to rebel. They secretly look for a way to cheat the system or deceive those who are seemingly in charge.

After losing 20 pounds, Debbie hit a weight plateau. In fact, her weight was starting to creep back up ever so slightly. As we talked about this, she told me she was starting to "rebel."

"That's an interesting way to put it," I said. "Tell me what you mean."

"Well, I know I have to follow this diet, and knowing I have to makes me want to do just the opposite," she said.

"Who said you had to follow the diet?"

"Well I guess no one actually said that." She broke eye contact and looked down at the table.

"Do you feel like our team is pressuring you?"

She leaned forward, placed her elbow on the table, and rested her head in her hand. "No, it's not you guys," she said as she ran her fingers side to side above her eyebrow.

"Debbie, you can do whatever you want. You're free to get up right now, head to Burger King, and order everything on the menu."

She giggled and then sighed. "I guess you're right, but it doesn't feel that way. I tell myself I have to do this. The more I tell myself I have to follow a diet and exercise, the less I want to do it. I start to rebel against my own thoughts. Am I crazy?"

Debbie was not crazy, but she was right about feeling rebellious because of her own thoughts. She made demands on herself that caused her to feel as if she didn't have a choice. Her compliant self was wagging a finger at her alter ego and saying, "You must eat this and you can't eat that." In response, the part of her that didn't like being told what to do was feeling the urge to flip her the bird, take her I'll-show-you attitude to a convenience store, and buy a candy bar and a regular, not diet, soda.

This back-and-forth type of thinking is not only exhausting, but can have a powerful effect on attitude—and our attitudes obviously impact our long-term behavior. The only way someone loses weight is to change behavior. We cannot educate our way to a healthier body, think our way to success, or pay our way to weight loss. In the end, it boils down to behavior: The types and amounts of food we eat and the physical activity we perform.

But focusing only on behavior is short-sighted when it comes to long-term weight management. Since most dieters already know about the behavior needed to lose weight, it makes sense to explore how our thoughts and feelings are connected to those behaviors. The following illustration shows that our thoughts, feelings, and behavior are connected, each influencing the other. The arrows between the three concepts are bi-directional which means that:

- Thinking can impact our behavior, and
- behavior can change our thinking.
- Thoughts can change our feelings, and
- our feelings impact our thoughts.
- Our feelings can affect behavior, similar to how
- behavior impacts our feelings.

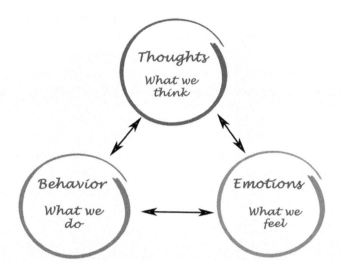

While working to become a better weight manager, you'll find it important to identify which of these connections most often gets in your way. Do you need a more structured behavior plan to improve your confidence? Or perhaps your plan is fine, but emotions derail your progress. Perhaps your thinking is the problem—how you interpret life situations leads to stress eating and abandoning your exercise routine.

Pete and Debbie showed us how thoughts, feelings, and behavior interact to shape our attitudes. The sections below provide specific examples of the six connections listed in the bullet points above. I encourage you to read each section with great attention and evaluate your strengths and weaknesses. This self-assessment will help you change your thoughts and set goals—topics you'll read about in upcoming chapters.

Emotions and Feelings—Not Exactly the Same

Although the circular illustration describes emotions as "something we feel," feelings and emotions aren't exactly the same. Emotions such as fear, anger, and happiness are unique physiological responses (responses that affect the body) and we're usually, but not always, aware of them. For example, with fear the body release stress hormones that can increase heart rate and breathing, along with other physical responses. Likewise with anger. When these are strong emotions, they're difficult to ignore. Happiness tells the brain to increase our energy level and suppress negative feelings. Sadness does the opposite.

Feelings are different. We're aware of feelings because that's how we describe what's happening to us internally — we *feel* bored or overwhelmed, for example. Psychologists often say that feelings are best described as your interpretation of an emotion.

> *Psychologists often say that feelings are best described as your interpretation of an emotion.*

For the purposes of weight management, you don't necessarily need to analyze whether you're experiencing an emotion or a feeling. But with some conditions, such as anxiety-related disorders, people often find it useful to distinguish between the two. In the sections that follow, I use the words *feelings* and *emotions* interchangeably.

The most important thing to understand is that feelings/emotions can result from, or lead to, thoughts and behavior. Therefore, they can help us, or interfere with, successful weight management.

Behavior Follows Thoughts

When patients describe *why* they overate or took a week off from exercise, I often hear about a *situation*. Maybe the person was traveling, working long hours, caring for a sick family member, or dealing with some other crisis. Just as 10-year old Emily said she ate tortilla chips because her dad bought them, many people tell me their circumstances caused their behavior. When they try to change behavior, they focus only on making the environment better or having more willpower when they can't change the circumstances. This flawed approach reminds me of a valuable lesson I learned from my mom.

When I was a preteen my mother would often say use "brains not brawn" when she saw me struggling to solve a mechanical issue like restringing a baseball glove or making a minor bike repair. When my solution involved brute force, she reminded me to think differently and strategize my approach. When I blamed the bike and tried to muscle my way through a solution, she was saying, "Slow down and think about the problem in a different way."

Just as Mom said, we also need to slow down and think differently to solve problems related to weight. Although changing a situation can be helpful, it isn't always possible or practical. Using *will power* isn't a sustainable solution either—will power is the brawn of behavior change. It can help at times, but that muscle is easily fatigued and we're left exhausted and frustrated by lack of success.

A more effective approach begins with increased awareness of how thoughts impact our behavior. Thoughts that turn into strong beliefs greatly influence our eating and physical activity. Many examples throughout this book have illustrated this—from Karen who viewed exercise as torture; to Rachel who viewed french fries as something that caused her to break out in fat like an allergic reaction; to folks like Pete who have a dry-drunk approach to dieting.

Our beliefs about the weight loss journey have a powerful impact on how we act and how easily we reach our goals for weight management. Behaving against our beliefs is hard work, like paddling upstream. Aligning our thoughts with healthy behavior allows us to lighten the load, places the wind at our backs, and helps us float downstream.

Unfortunately, we don't always recognize when underlying thoughts and beliefs are shaping our eating and exercise habits. An eating binge can start from thoughts about a seemingly unrelated situation that makes you feel frustrated. One client told me that when she was growing up, her family blew the smallest problems out of proportion. Their motto for dealing with these situations was, "The sky is falling, let's eat cake!" Thoughts about something unrelated to eating—a car that needed unexpected repair or a broken pair of glasses, ended up leading to unhealthy eating. Their mountain-out-of-a-mole-hill thoughts led to seeking food for calm and comfort. For this family, thoughts did not directly impact behavior. Instead, thoughts about their situation led to negative feelings. These negative feelings led them to turn to food (thoughts-feelings-behavior).

> *Mountain-out-of-a-molehill thinking can lead to seeking food for calm and comfort*

Sometimes Behavior Leads the Way to Healthier Thinking

Although you just read that getting your mind right is essential for long-term success, we can't always wait for the perfect perspective before getting started with weight management. Changing our behavior can become the first step while working to get thoughts totally on board.

Like many of the people I've worked with, Judy tried for years to lose weight. She had a pattern of dropping 20 or 30 pounds only to regain it, plus a little more, with each attempt. When we met she was 100 pounds heavier than when she married 27 years earlier. After years of failure, her confidence in her ability to lose weight and keep it off had reached an all-time low. When several of her co-workers had successful weight loss after bariatric surgery, Judy wondered if surgery would work for her. This glimmer of hope led to an appointment with her family physician to discuss the procedure. She contacted her insurance company, had the required psychological evaluation, and prepared for surgery by beginning to change her diet, take vitamins, and start a regular routine of physical activity. Despite her preparation and excitement, Judy had doubts that she would succeed in the long run. She knew she could lose weight for three or four months, but keeping it off seemed impossible.

Although Judy was filled with self-doubt, sprinkled with a bit of hope, surgery day arrived and she didn't back out. In fact, after surgery she attended all her postoperative appointments and followed the recommended eating plan. In some ways the surgery *forced* certain behavior changes; she could only eat small portions and the smell of certain foods she used to enjoy made her nauseous. In just six months she reached a weight she hadn't seen since before she became pregnant with her oldest son 16 years earlier. Her knee pain lessened, she stopped her blood pressure medicine, and her husband told her she no longer snored.

Despite her success, Judy was still fearful. She'd never kept weight off this long and wondered if she would start regaining, even though her now tangerine-sized stomach limited food intake and her appetite wasn't what it used to be. Even though she had doubts, she continued to make all her appointments with the registered dietitian and worked hard to follow the agreed-upon goals. Soon she reached her one-year surgery anniversary and was starting to believe she could actually succeed. The longer she followed the plan, the more confident she became. Judy's story had a happy ending as success bred success, with her behavior leading the way.

> *Sometimes our thoughts lag behind our behavior, and that's okay.*

Judy's success illustrates that sometimes our thoughts lag behind our behavior, and that's okay. Even when thinking isn't quite where it needs to be, a realistic plan, accountability, support, and a commitment to "stay in the game" can lead to short-term success. The longer this success lasts, the more our confidence grows, leading to a change in mindset. As Judy embraced her new body and abilities she was more likely to join a walking group, make friends with similar health interests, and take up hobbies that weren't centered on eating. With each positive change the chances of relapsing into her old lifestyle diminished.

Although we should always try to get our minds ready for behavior changes, weight management can be sort of like having kids. If potential parents waited until they were one hundred percent ready, humans would never reproduce. When it comes to weight, sometimes we have to make the leap, knowing our thoughts can evolve—especially if we're intentional about addressing them along the way.

The Connection between Behavior and Emotions

Dogs quickly learn that leashes are awesome. You put the leash on Max, pet him feverishly, tell him he's a good boy in a strange voice, and head out the door for a walk. Once he learns this pattern, even the rattle of a leash brings him running to you, tail wagging. Why do dogs react this way? They learn the leash means positive attention, plus they get to go outside and smell everything in the neighborhood. The way humans become emotionally attached to eating isn't much different from Max's love for his leash.

I learned this firsthand as a child—with my grandmother. She lived next door to us and often expressed her love for me by making delicious buttermilk biscuits. When spending the night with her I'd fall asleep looking forward to breakfast the next morning. I can still visualize every step of the biscuit making.

Still wearing her housecoat, my grandmother sifted Gold Medal flour through a dented tin sifter. Her thin hands worked in the shortening and then poured the buttermilk into the bowl. She talked to me, rarely looking down at the work in front of her, as she effortlessly rolled the biscuits in oil and neatly placed them side-by-side in a large cast-iron skillet that used to be her mother's. Similar to Max's excitement when his owner brought the leash, watching Grandma prepare food filled me with anticipation and positive feelings.

I believe Grandma enjoyed those mornings as much as I did. She loved to tease me by saying she didn't know if she could remember how to "make a good pan" anymore. At her recent funeral I learned that her mother (my great grandmother) would bake three dozen biscuits every morning to feed the 13 children in their country home in Mississippi. They were poor, but well loved, and the daily biscuits were fit for a king—just like my grandma's. Because of her own upbringing, baking biscuits meant something to her, and she passed along this family tradition to me. In a sense, her biscuits were like an always-fresh heirloom, golden and slightly crisp on the outside, with fluffy buttermilk goodness on the inside.

When I was upset about losing a baseball game or tired from the grind of elementary school, Grandma baked a pan of biscuits for me. They symbolized her love and were often just what I needed to make my simple world a little bit brighter. To this day I think of her whenever I use a cast-iron skillet. Her dented sifter sits in my cabinet, often bringing a smile to my face or occasional tears to my eyes. I don't often eat biscuits, but when I do, I think of Grandma, because I have an emotional attachment to this particular food.

Just like me, you probably have strong emotional connections to certain foods. These are often cultural, related to childhood, and can be evoked by sight, sound, and especially smell. Unfortunately, most of us aren't emotionally attached to green, leafy foods. We remember things like mom's macaroni and cheese, warm homemade pie with ice cream, birthday cake, pizza, and many other delightful foods. When we eat them, the food not only tastes good, but brings back happy memories, like turning the pages of a family album.

If these connections are strong enough and you don't have other, healthier ways to meet your emotional needs, you may find yourself using comfort foods to relieve boredom, fight off loneliness, or ease the pain of a hurtful comment or toxic relationship.

> *You may find yourself using comfort foods to relieve boredom, fight off loneliness, or ease the pain of a hurtful comment or toxic relationship.*

For some people emotions are not tied to a certain food, but to eating in general. This type of emotional eating can be related to escaping negative experiences. Childhood trauma commonly triggers the use of food for distraction and comfort—stuffing down those bad memories with a bag of potato chips or a pint of ice cream.

In severe cases, eating can become part of dissociation from reality. A patient once described her escape-from-life binges as so intense that the edges of tortilla chips left her upper mouth full of cuts. Another patient described a failed attempt to stop her binge eating when she dug food out of her trash can after throwing it away to stop the behavior. Both of these clients had experienced traumatic events which influenced them to develop this pattern of emotional eating. Their stories, like those of many of my clients, were difficult to listen to. The mistreatment wasn't their fault and food had evolved into something much more than nourishment and pleasure. People with this type of connection to food will likely need the help of a skilled therapist to recover—and recovery is possible.

More commonly, people describe checking out with food that is not as intense. Perhaps you may mindlessly consume food because you're using it as an emotion regulator while your attention is elsewhere. A former colleague told me she was once eating a bag of chips while nervously cramming for an exam at The University of New Orleans. She wasn't even looking at the food she was scooping out of the bag when out of the corner of her eye she noticed a large palmetto bug trapped in the middle of a handful of chips she was about to stuff into her mouth. By the way, a palmetto bug is a nice word Southerners use for "cockroach."

> *When emotions are coupled with eating we can form strong and often unhealthy connections between the two.*

When emotions are coupled with eating we can form strong and often unhealthy connections between the two. This obviously has an impact on weight. Similarly, we can form healthy or unhealthy emotion-behavior connections that impact physical activity and help or hinder our weight loss efforts. A number of people have described terrible experiences in gym class that later triggered negative memories and emotions. When they think of exercise, they remember the teachers who embarrassed them in front of their classmates or the kids who made fun of their bodies in the locker room. Maybe your emotional reaction stems from feeling singled out as you finished minutes behind the next-to-last student running laps.

Some people were punished with exercise in school, sports, or the military. Doing push-ups or running laps to atone for mistakes does little to foster a love for physical activity. By comparison, others have fond memories of riding bikes as a family, playing little league baseball or softball, soccer, or hiking. They view exercise as enjoyable and fulfilling rather than threatening and punishing.

Are These Connections Permanent?

It's okay if you have certain emotional connections with food you don't want to change. I hope biscuits will always remind me of Grandma. But as you know by now, too many emotion-food associations will jeopardize your health. The good news is: If your behavior and emotions surrounding food are linked in unhealthy ways, they don't have to stay that way.

Through a process psychologists call counterconditioning, we can get rid of unhealthy connections and replace them with healthier ones.

For instance, we tend to feel happy during celebrations, holidays, and vacations. Rather than coupling these positive emotions with unhealthy foods and inactivity, we can create more healthy connections. Making fresh fruit (rather than lots of cake and ice cream) part of summer birthday celebrations and walking in a local Turkey Trot (to replace the tradition of baking cinnamon rolls) every Thanksgiving morning with your family can become enjoyable traditions. Relaxing, fun-filled vacations can include hiking, walking on the beach and preparing meals together. Once we're accustomed to this, we may find these trips more enjoyable than outings filled with excessive drinking, overeating at restaurants, and inactivity. If snow means having a good time sledding (instead of a cookie and hot chocolate fest) and hot weather means swimming (rather than hotdogs and lemonade) we begin to strengthen the connection between health, exercise, and positive emotions.

Feelings Can Impact Thinking

We all have days when we "wake up on the wrong side of the bed." For some reason, our mood just isn't bright. Maybe we're a little sleep deprived; perhaps it's hormonal (such as premenstrual syndrome) or related to neurotransmitter reuptake in our brain (depression). For other people, these feelings are wrapped in a dark cloud of chronic pain. One thing is sure, when we *feel* a certain way, our thoughts are almost sure to follow.

Much of the time, especially when I'm full of energy and in a good mood, I know how lucky I am to have children. I want to savor every moment with them, knowing I'll never see them at this exact age ever again. I'm thankful they're healthy and can be rambunctious and ornery. I appreciate their budding personalities, innocence, and unrelenting desire to learn about the world around them. My 5-year-old daughter's animal sounds are sort of cute and I love that my 6-year-old son wants me to multiply 800 zillion by 22 million, two hundred thirty-seven. But when I'm exhausted, things are different. I'm almost ashamed to admit it, but those animal sounds can be really annoying. And how many times have I told my son that zillion isn't really a number? Fatigue easily leads to frustration about their disobedience. "Do other kids really act like this?" "Why does everything they touch become sticky, greasy, or leave a pile of debris behind?"

They're like tornadoes tearing through the house and I wish I could just wave a wand and their faces would be washed, teeth brushed, and they would be expert butt-wipers without any parental assistance. During these times, I know that fatigue has influenced my thoughts.

The depth of our experiences and responses to emotion is one thing separating humans from other mammals. Fits of rage, panic, and severe depression can leave us wondering if a simpler brain might be better. Sometimes it's easy to look at the dog and think, "Max, you've got it made. As long as somebody feeds you, pets you occasionally and lets you run around peeing wherever you want, you seem pretty content with life." On the other hand, our ability to fall head over heels in love with someone or laugh so hard we cry is a wonderful part of being human. Just like anything with more power and complexity, our brains allow us to experience extreme emotions. Since emotion is closely tied to behavior (such as eating), it's essential for each of us to understand emotion-provoked thought patterns. People who ignore their thoughts and feelings usually don't succeed with weight management in the long run.

> *People who ignore their thoughts and feelings usually don't succeed with weight management in the long run.*

Vicious Circle or Roadmap?

The triad of emotion, thoughts, and beliefs we've looked at can turn into a vicious circle or become a helpful map to successful weight management. In the upcoming chapters we'll explore how specific thought patterns can help or hinder your progress.

Chapter 9

The Bad Smell of Stinkin' Thinkin'

IN THIS SECTION we're exploring how the relationship of thoughts, feelings, and behavior affects our eating and exercise habits. In this chapter, thinking takes center stage.

Before we get started let's clarify a few concepts and terms. Each of us has thoughts we can't entirely control. Sometimes we know certain thoughts are ridiculous and we can easily dismiss them and ask ourselves, "Where did that come from?" We won't be scrutinizing those thoughts. Instead, I want to focus on thoughts that matter—the ones that influence behavior and shape our attitudes and beliefs.

Beliefs are simply thoughts we accept as true. If your mind was a garden, thoughts would be seeds that quickly developed into seedlings. Beliefs and attitudes are the mature plants. Therefore, thoughts are full of potential to help us and provide a sense of well-being. Too often, however, they derail us—and that's where this chapter can help. Let's look at three clients whose thinking directly affected their attempts at weight loss:

- John needed to make changes in his diet before being approved for bariatric surgery. As I explained the MyPlate principles of healthy eating, John snapped back at me, "I'm not doing that. Nobody eats that way!"

- A client named Karmen told me her personal trainer said she was obese because she'd ruined her metabolism. According to him, regular, intense workouts were the only way to solve her weight problem.

- Becky's mother always told her she'd never find a *good man* if she was overweight. Now 32 years old, 75 pounds overweight, and still single—Becky felt unlovable.

Can you see how John, Karmen, and Becky handicapped their weight management efforts before they even started? John's belief that only freaks would eat a balanced diet was like putting up a huge DETOUR sign on the road to weight loss. Karmen was overwhelmed by thinking her metabolism was forever ruined and only a lifelong extreme exercise program would treat her condition. She was bound to give up. Becky's mother primed her to feel lonely and hopeless in pursuit of a relationship. She quickly dismissed any man who showed interest in her, yet paid close attention if anyone seemed put off by her weight. Eating would become her friend, her solace.

These three examples above show how thinking can have a clear, direct relationship to weight. However, sometimes the beliefs that affect eating and physical activity are more subtle and indirect:

- At work, Steve's philosophy was, "If *I* don't do this, it won't get done" At the same time, he had high standards for work and wouldn't delegate tasks to others. This led to 14-hour days with no time for exercise. Being strapped for time and chronically sleep deprived, he often ordered carry-out and drank caffeinated sugar-sweetened beverages all day long.

- For years Sarah tried not to even think about her family, but she couldn't get them out of her mind. Her alcoholic father's relapse made her both angry and sad. Her sister's lifestyle choices led to financial problems, and Sarah felt obligated to help. Sarah seemed to always feel upset, and to keep those emotions under control she distracted herself in some way—often by eating something she knew she shouldn't.

- Lisa often thought about how terrible it would be if she disappointed her boss, her husband, or her kids. She believed she needed to be everything for everyone, and this led to anxiety she couldn't control. She felt anxious much of the time and eating became her Xanax.

The First Steps toward Change

The first step toward thinking differently is to recognize beliefs and feelings behind the behavior we want to change. Examining situations and their outcome helps pinpoint our problematic behavior. For example, let's consider Lisa from the last paragraph and imagine how she might respond to the following scenario:

Lisa's boss asks for a volunteer to lead a fundraising project (situation). Lisa thinks, "My boss will be disappointed in me if I don't do it" (thought) and despite her already overcommitted schedule, she feels pressure (emotion/feeling) to take on the task. For Lisa, this becomes a question of which option is most unpleasant: the anxiety of not volunteering versus the anxiety and stress of accepting extra work she doesn't want. Either way, she feels stressed because her thinking has created a lose-lose situation.

Lisa could think differently: "I'm not sure what my boss expects, but even if he does want me to do this (and I have no evidence that he does), it's unreasonable for me to be everything for everybody. Other people in the office can benefit from taking a turn. The people who truly care about me will still feel that way even if I don't always do exactly what they want." She could also talk to her boss in private about his expectations. Thinking differently helps Lisa feel less anxious about her situation. Her new thinking may feel awkward at first but allows her to make the brave choice of saying "no" to more responsibility.

The ABC's of thinking

A simple process can help people like Lisa change their thinking. Based on the work of Albert Ellis and Aaron Beck, cognitive behavioral therapy includes identifying a situation (activating event) that leads to a thought/belief, that in turn yields an emotional reaction. In Lisa's case the process looked like this:

Activating Event (A): Boss asks for a volunteer.

Belief (B): "The boss will be disappointed if I don't volunteer."

Consequence (C): Feeling pressured, overwhelmed, and even angry.

A simple ABC process can help us identify and change unproductive thoughts.

Patients come to see me to lose weight. But my patients don't lose weight before every visit. Sometimes they gain quite a bit, depending on how long they've been away and events in their lives. Body language usually reveals their expectations even before they step onto the scale. Patients who know their weight is up are sometimes tearful, disgusted with themselves, and embarrassed. After a weight check, our interaction might go something like this:

"You seem upset, what's going on?"

"It's just that my weight is up. I'm so frustrated."

"Were you expecting it to be up?"

"Yeah, I guess, but seeing it reminds me that I'm not reaching my goals."

"So you're upset because you feel like you're not making any progress right now?"

Weight gain is the activating event here. Patients tell me they're upset by the added pounds, but that is actually *not* why they're upset. They are unhappy because of **beliefs** about increased weight. If gaining weight automatically caused distress, then *everyone* who added a few pounds would be unhappy. Yet, weight gain is often desirable for people who are too thin. Therefore, seeing numbers go up on a scale isn't guaranteed to cause unhappiness. Our personal **beliefs** about weight gain inspire feelings like these:

"I'm hopeless at losing weight."

"This diet and exercise thing isn't going to work for me."

"People are laughing at me."

These beliefs—not the actual weight gain—lead to the **consequence** of negative feelings. And those negative feelings make us want to give up, which would create even more emotional distress.

Activating Event (A): Gained 10 pounds.

Belief (B): "I have absolutely no willpower."

Consequence (C): Feeling frustrated, angry, and hopeless. Tempted to stop trying.

You may be asking, "How can I think more positively if my weight gain was caused by ignoring my goals, emotional eating, or late-night snacking? In these instances, we are not necessarily looking for *positive* thoughts, but instead rational, functional thoughts that can help you get back on track. We want to think in a way that's functional without making it personal and judgmental.

Instead of using beliefs to put yourself down, translate your beliefs into rational, functional thoughts that will help you move forward without overwhelming blame and shame.

Activating Event: Gained 10 pounds.

Belief: For me, snacking late at night leads to weight gain. But I can control this behavior with a reasonable plan.

Consequence: I feel hopeful and will plan my snacks this week.

Thoughts Are Automatic

The bad thing about dysfunctional thinking is that our thoughts are often automatic. We respond to a situation in the same way for so long that the situation-thought-emotion cycle becomes like a bad golf swing repeated over and over for years; it seems almost impossible to change. We begin telling ourselves, "That's just how I think. It's part of my personality." Even if we want to think differently, those knee-jerk-reaction thoughts keep popping up and we don't even realize the damage they're doing until we've lashed out at someone, checked out with three glasses of wine, or polished off a bag of Ruffles. The thoughts are as automatic as flipping on a light switch even after you've lost power in your house.

We could compare the brain's neural networks to a daily commute. Perhaps you've taken the same morning drive for fifteen years, which includes traveling the same roads and encountering familiar traffic lights, merges, and landmarks. This daily routine is a highly organized schema in our mind and requires little thought or processing. You can do it on autopilot and barely remember the trip after you arrive. Even if the streets are congested and dangerous you take them anyway, because it's the only path available, or is the most reasonable option to take you where you need to go. But what if you discovered a newly constructed road that was safer, required less time, and was more scenic? Would you take it? I'm guessing you would, but you'd need to be intentional about the choice. If you forgot to focus on the new route, in a morning stupor you might still drive the old way.

Sometimes change requires great effort. Our home is in a newly developed neighborhood and the builder piled huge mounds of dirt in an empty lot about 50 yards behind our property. We could see the pile of dirt from the sunroom of the back of our house and of course my children wanted this to be their new playground. So I checked it out and decided they were unlikely to become *permanently* maimed by playing there.

I spoke to my wife about letting the little ankle biters expend some energy playing "King of the World" and "Mountain Tag," and she agreed, as long as it happened before their baths. We still had one problem: The only reasonable trek to this alluring dirt pile meant walking to the front of our house, along the road, and then along a dirt path created by the builder where work trucks frequently traveled. From inside our house we couldn't see our preschoolers walk this way, and even if we could see them, we didn't feel the route was safe without adult supervision. So if they wanted to play, my wife or I needed to chaperone them to the pile. This round-about trek was a major inconvenience because as soon as we reached the dirt pile one child needed to go to the bathroom or was hungry and wanted to come back to the house, and then back to the mountain—and back—and forth.

If only the kids could just walk out the back door and run safely to the dirt pile. We could keep an eye on them from the rear of our house and easily hear what was happening. But the landscape in between included high weeds, sticker bushes, and insects. I even saw a small garter snake back there. The weeds were so high we'd lose sight of our kids if they tried to hike through them. Besides, a previous attempt led to ouchies, bug bites, and a quick return to our backyard after four steps into the tangled mess of vegetation. After a weekend of walking the kids back and forth to the dirt pile via the road, I decided we had to find a better way.

I got out a hatchet and begin cutting down the weeds and brush that separated our backyard from the dirt pile. With the big stuff out of the way, I took our push mower and began making a path. The mosquitos were terrible and my mower wasn't made to cut tall weeds, but with persistence I eventually reached the dirt pile. The kids now had a safe, short, and efficient route to their playground that didn't require hand-holding.

Our thoughts are sometimes like the first route my kids first took to the dirt pile. They cause anxiety, are inefficient, and require a lot of support from others in order to make them work in our daily lives. Changing these entrenched thoughts often requires the tough work of creating a new set of beliefs and different neural pathways in the brain. This can take determination and, like making a path to the mountain, it requires tools and persistence.

One of the first steps to changing your thinking is to identify thoughts that get in your way. Categorizing these irrational beliefs can lead to building a shortcut that will bypass the weeds and lead directly to functional thinking and healthier behavior.

All or Nothing Thinking

For just a moment, think about the first Monday of January. This is the day when people return to work and school after the holidays. Those who vowed to get in shape this year set their alarms early to nudge their bodies onto the treadmill or to the nearest gym. For many, this is the first day of their "diet." Radio, TV, and the Internet are flooded with advertisements for weight loss programs and products. Many people who went to bed as late-night snacking slugs hope to awaken in the morning as die-hard dedicated dieters and fitness fanatics.

This type of all-or-nothing behavior is great for the 60 billion dollar per year weight-loss industry because, in addition to first time customers, companies depend on restarts. The restarts are the people who join another program, buy an additional piece of exercise equipment, join a different gym, purchase another book, or hire a personal trainer. Often these consumers are declaring their "all in" mentality. This is the year they will change—just like last year, and the year before that.

Motivation, drive, and excitement can be instrumental in helping us accomplish important goals such as losing weight.

But when we look at things in a polarized way, we end up repeating cycles of weight loss and regain. Whether related to health or other aspects of our lives, this all-or-nothing thinking can be frustrating, inefficient, and even catastrophic. Can you imagine what life would be like if people took the all-or-nothing approach to driving? Some days people would drive under the speed limit, stop at red lights, and yield to pedestrians, but on other days they'd ignore all traffic laws — sort of like downtown Boston.

In reality, most of our behavior is on a continuum, even if our thinking isn't. For example, if you think someone is a terrible person that thought can easily become a belief that will impact how you respond to him or her. Although you probably won't *behave* in an all-or-nothing way (hugging versus physically harming), your all-or-nothing thoughts (great person versus terrible person) have a significant effect on interactions. You certainly won't go out of your way to know this person better.

When we think, "I'm either on a diet or out of control," our behavior is likely to drift in that direction as well. Here's an example of three all-or-nothing thoughts that might impact your eating and physical activity.

- *If I don't stay under my calorie goal I have failed.*
- *If I can't get my heart rate up for 30 minutes, then exercise does me no good.*
- *I have no self-control when it comes to sweets; once I get started I can't stop.*

Let's look at these thoughts. What happens if we believe the first example? Does that mean if you're one calorie over the goal you have totally failed?   Do you get discouraged at this point and perhaps overeat even more?

If you believe exercise is only useful if it's intense for 30 minutes, how often will you miss the opportunity for a 10-minute walk that will reduce stress? How often will you ignore the benefits of exercising during TV commercials?

Is it really true that once you get started on sweets you can't stop? Does this happen in all situations, no matter what?

Sherry's problem was salty, crunchy, fatty foods. She told me potato chips were the worst, or best, depending on how you look at it.

"If I have one, I eat until they're all gone," she told me.

"That happens every time?" I asked.

She shrugged. "Pretty much."

Coincidentally, our weight management center was conducting research on preferences for regular versus baked potato chips during this time, so we had a stockpile of both kinds in the office.

"Hang on a minute, I want to test your theory," I told Sherry.

I went to the back and filled a Styrofoam bowl with the regular, full-fat chips. I placed the bowl of chips in front of Sherry and said, "I want to try something with you."

With a here-comes-a-magic-trick expression on her face, she agreed.

"I want you to eat a chip," I said.

Sherry smiled, selected the largest chip, and willingly crunched, chewed and swallowed. Then I waited. I looked at Sherry in anticipation of her next move. Finally, she got a little uncomfortable.

"What?"

"Aren't you going to eat the rest of them?" I asked.

"No."

"Why not?"

With an uncomfortable laugh, she said, "Because you're here!"

"If I leave the room, will you eat the rest of them?"

"Nooo."

"What about on your way home, will you stop and buy more?" I asked.

"No, I don't think so," Sherry said smiling.

"So it really isn't true that once you eat one chip you can't stop?"

"Well, I usually eat chips at home in front of the TV. I take the whole bag to the couch and before I know it, they're all gone."

"So when you eat chips in *that* sort of environment it's hard to control yourself?"

"Exactly."

Sherry's belief that she couldn't stop eating chips once she started wasn't true. In fact, she could practice a lot of restraint in certain settings. She had options with potato chips. She didn't need to accept the idea that they controlled her. Instead, if she wanted to eat chips in moderation, she could set up her environment to increase the likelihood for success. Maybe she could buy a vending machine size bag, or pre-portion her chips into smaller containers. She could commit to only eating chips at the kitchen table where she could truly pay attention to the pleasure from one serving. Or, she could only eat chips when she came to her weight management appointments. Lastly, Sherry might decide that keeping chips in the house was just too much work and the chips weren't worth it. Whatever she decided, the crucial element was believing she could control herself—and we proved that during our session with the chips.

Countless other all-or-nothing thoughts can impact eating, such as:

- I totally blew it by oversleeping, missing my workout, and then skipping breakfast. No use trying to get back on track today.

- My presentation was a total disaster.

- Yesterday was great, but today has been the worst.

- I either avoid carbs altogether or I'm eating chips and cookies.

- Nobody cares anything about me unless they're getting something from me.

- My husband always ignores my needs; it's all about him, never about me.

- It's either organic vegetables or no vegetables at all.

Whether the thought is about the weight loss process itself or another area of your life, it can impact your health behavior. If you're so distraught by your *worst day ever* at your job that you can't stomach the idea of going home, preparing dinner, and cleaning up the mess, you may end up ordering a pizza. If you feel *nobody* cares about you and your life is without purpose, why bother taking care of yourself?

This all-or-nothing thinking is one of many thought patterns that can get in our way, and we're going to look at options to combat it. But first, let's examine other categories of thinking that derail us.

Filter-Focus

A friend of mine used to say, "Filter-focus!" when saw a good-looking guy who grabbed her attention. She would fan herself as she repeated the phrase *filter-focus, filter-focus*. Her objective was to filter out thoughts about him so she could focus on what she was doing.

At any given moment we're bombarded by information from at least four of our five senses. As children we're easily distracted and don't always filter and focus well. For instance, kids may dart into traffic when they see something interesting. But as we learn and our brains mature, we become better at filtering out a tremendous amount of data by prioritizing. This mostly happens "behind the scenes" without our awareness. This filtering activity often affects our attitudes and behavior.

Depending on our personality and experiences, we can learn to filter out information—or we can prioritize it in ways that cause unnecessary and harmful stress.

Some people filter out accomplishments and focus only on their deficiencies, especially those related to weight. An example would be ignoring the two pounds you lost, while focusing on a package of cookies you ate this morning. This viewpoint leads down a road of frustration and hopelessness, paved with the perceived tragedy of many failures. Don't get me wrong, we do need to understand and evaluate our mishaps, but only if we also enjoy our positive attributes and success.

Filter-focus fallacy can expand to include our overall moods and life perspective. Choosing to mainly focus on the positive aspects of life changes your outlook on every situation, the people you encounter, and yourself. If you're accustomed to negativity, the idea of changing to a positive focus may seem "soft" and unrealistic. "The world is a hard place," these people say. "Better get used to it."

Yes, bad things happen all around us—but what about the good stuff? If you let your mind process life according to the nightly news, you won't feel uplifted or positive toward your own life and the people around you. School shootings, murder, scandals, politicians verbally attacking each other, traffic congestion, and impending bad weather, slightly tempered with a sprinkle of a feel-good story or humor—that's the news, every day. If we want to experience joy, we should avoid seeing our lives from a nightly-news perspective. Furthermore, if we want to stay committed to healthy living, we cannot filter out our achievements and focus only on failures.

When I review a food journal with someone who has filter-focus problems, the conversation often goes something like this:

"Thanks for letting me take a look at this. You did a nice job of consistently tracking your food. Tell me a little bit about what went well and what you're still struggling with."

"Well, I'm still snacking too much at night and I know I need to eat breakfast every day, but I don't. This week has been terrible for exercise because I've been working more and I'm just so tired when I get home."

"Ok, but you did eat breakfast four times this week, which is an improvement, and I notice you're taking your lunch a bit more instead of going out to eat."

"Yeah, but I'm still eating out too much. I want to get out of the office, and when my co-workers suggest it, I go. I just don't seem to have much willpower when it comes to lunch, especially on the days when I skip breakfast."

"I understand you still want to make improvements, but over the past several weeks you've been moving in that direction. What do you think you did well that led to you losing weight?"

"Well I'm just kicking myself right now because I wanted to lose five pounds in two weeks and I only lost three. I need to dedicate myself much more to exercise and sticking closer to the plan."

Despite promptings, this patient could not give herself credit for her accomplishments. If you've ever been involved with someone who filtered out your accomplishments and focused on your imperfections, you understand the consequences. No matter what you do it isn't good enough, and if you succeed at something they remind you of previous failures with statements like these:

"I wish you'd done that a long time ago, I don't know why it took you so long to figure it out."

"I see you made the honor roll, but why did you get a 'B' in that class. Were you goofing off?"

"Your sales figures topped everyone else's this month, but you should aim higher than that."

"If you people really cared about this project you'd be working more overtime."

Do comments like this motivate you to do your best? Do they spur you on? I doubt it. Instead you feel beaten down. The joy of accomplishment is easily squashed, and after a while you think, "Why bother? Nothing I do will be good enough."

When we talk to ourselves in the same way, the same feelings emerge. The other harmful aspect of filter-focus is that constructive criticism is no longer effective. When you or someone else finds fault with everything you do, one criticism becomes just like all of the others. On the other hand, when you're able to focus on what you've done well you're more likely to appreciate a valid critique.

Mind Reading

Assuming we know what other people are thinking can get us into big trouble. This fallacy of thought can fuel racism, perpetuate neighborhood feuds, lead to social anxiety, result in road rage, and contribute to disintegrating marriages. When we try to read another person's mind we're often wrong—but we act on those beliefs anyway. If my wife lets me oversleep because she knows I'm extra tired, I might "read her mind" and decide she let me oversleep to prove a point about my inability to set an alarm. This could lead to an argument over nothing.

The hard part about mind reading is *sometimes* we get it right, which reminds us to keep doing it. We remember the times we assumed correctly and tend to forget the times we guessed wrong.

Mind reading can obstruct weight management by causing anxiety and concern over what others think about us. Thinking this way can result in self-imposed pressure to prove something to a boss, sibling, spouse, or co-worker. As a result we may eat to help relieve the stress caused by these feelings—or we may lose focus on weight-related goals.

Mind reading can *directly* impact health behavior if we make assumptions about what others think about our size, what we eat, or our competence using exercise equipment at the gym.

At our initial session I had asked Tara if she'd be willing to keep a food journal so we could review it a week later. As we began our second session, I asked how things had gone the previous week. Tara was polite but a bit jittery as we sat three feet apart with a round table between us. Every minute or so she pulled at the front of her shirt to prevent it from conforming to the body she'd grown to hate. She had kept a food and activity journal using an app on her phone, but it remained tucked in her purse, which was on the floor near her feet. As I began to ask specific questions about eating and exercise, she again picked at her shirt.

"I know you're going to think this is just an excuse but we had out-of-town guests this week and I didn't follow the plan very well."

As I tried to reassure her that my role was to help, not judge, I asked if I could take a look at her food journal. She leaned over, picked up her large purse, and began to rifle through it.

"You must think I'm really disorganized. I know my phone is in here," she said. Finally she pulled out the phone and a crumpled tissue fell on the table. "I'm sorry, that's embarrassing."

"It's okay, really—if I had a purse I can only imagine what might fall out of it," I said, hoping to help her feel at ease.

She quickly stuffed the tissue back in her purse and set the phone near her body at the edge of the table. She looked down at her phone, rubbing her thumb back and forth on the screen trying to clean it.

"Before you look at this, I just want you to know that I'm not lazy and I know I shouldn't eat this way. I'm sure all of you guys eat well and exercise—but I'm just not there yet. You probably think I'm not going to do well because I've already messed up and it's only the first week of the program."

"Tara, I honestly haven't made any assumptions about you and how you're going to do in the program." I paused, hoping she would look up from her phone. When she didn't, I gently placed my hand flat on the table only inches from her. I leaned forward and tilted my head to the side in hopes of lifting her gaze toward me. She looked up. "I'm just glad you're here and willing to allow me to work with you on some of the things you're struggling with. I assure you, none of *our* diets are perfect and nobody exercises every day for months on end," I said, before I pulled my hand back to my side of the table. "If you don't want me to look at your food journal right now that's okay. We can do that some other time."

Tara took a deep breath and then agreed to let me see the records. She logged into her app and handed me her phone. She squirmed in her chair and quickly pulled her shirt away from her body.

Tara's anxiety was clearly related to mind reading. She made assumptions about what I believed about her and that would interfere with treatment until I, and the rest of the team, could establish trust. I've worked with many people who think like Tara—people who won't go to a gym or walk outside because they *know* what others will think of their size; or clients who practice tremendous restraint with eating around others because of similar fears of what people will think if they see an overweight person eating something unhealthy. Of course this restraint can't be maintained, and when the person is alone the wheels fall off.

The fact of the matter is: We don't know what others are thinking. To be honest, at times I don't even know what I'm thinking myself. Things tend to jostle around in my head like a pinball machine. If I can't tell you exactly what *I'm* thinking, how can someone *else* know what's going on inside my head?

One way to deal with mind reading is to simply let go of assumptions. By definition, an assumption means you don't have proof to support your belief. You are guessing. Is it really worth getting worked up over a guess? Another approach is to broaden your speculations about what others are thinking by using a variety of *may* statements. When we expand our guess it's important to include opposing perspectives. If your mind reading keeps you from the gym because you believe people think you don't belong there, you might tell yourself: "The buffed up guy may be thinking I don't know what I'm doing, or he may be thinking *way to go*, or he may be thinking about the size of his biceps and have no idea I'm even around."

> *An assumption means you don't have proof to support a belief. You are guessing. Is it really worth it to get worked up over a guess?*

Catastrophic Predictions

"If I don't lose weight now, I never will."

"Really? Why do you say that? I asked."

"My doctor told me I'm no longer pre-diabetic; I actually *have* diabetes. My knees hurt and I take six different medications every day. If that isn't enough motivation, nothing will ever get my butt in gear."

The idea that you'll never lose weight if you don't do it now is a good example of a catastrophic prediction. This way of thinking creates enormous pressure to change. Although this pressure can yield results in the short run, it doesn't work well as a long-term perspective. A now-or-never mindset builds resentment and is emotionally exhausting. You may believe that putting intense pressure on yourself to change NOW will eventually lead to healthy habits. But our minds don't work that way. Think about anything you were pressured to do as a child (play a sport, take piano lessons). If you didn't begin enjoying yourself or grasp its value early in the process, you probably fizzled out before long. As we will discuss later, choice is much easier to sustain than pressure.

> *A now-or-never mindset builds resentment and is emotionally exhausting.*

Catastrophic predictions in other areas of our lives also create anxiety. The single mom in the inner city may believe that if her child doesn't do his homework every single night he'll end up on drugs or in prison. This thought process causes her to feel anxious, and as a result of her fear, she pressures her son over doing homework. Her approach is not calm and supportive, but instead demanding and authoritarian. Unfortunately, this method probably won't yield a happy homework time or a love of academic pursuits for her son— unless she can also instill in him the value of an education.

Labeling

"So Bob, tell me why you've had trouble getting into a regular exercise routine."

"That's an easy question. I'm just lazy."

Lightheartedly, I responded, "Well, I have to be honest with you—I can't fix lazy! Let me ask you a few other questions. You have a job, right?"

Bob nods his head, "Yep, two more years 'til I can retire."

"Kids?"

"Three of them, and all out of the house. I've got two grandkids thanks to my oldest son and his wife."

"Do you get to spend much time with your grandkids?"

Bob leaned back in his chair and chuckled. "They live nearby and it's one of the greatest pleasures in my life. I take my 7-year-old grandson fishing almost every weekend in the summer. My 4-year-old granddaughter—now she's a piece of work—she likes to come over and ride on the tractor with me."

"So they love spending time with their grandpa!"

"Oh, you betcha," he leaned forward as though telling me a secret. "Last time after they were over they asked their mom if they could move in with us." Bob sat back and pushed his glasses back towards his face. "I guess we'd have room. Heck we have ten acres, we could build on if we wanted!"

"It sounds like there's a lot to take care of at home. Do you mow most of the land?"

"I mow about two acres, the rest is just woods—my granddaughter would tell you she mows the yard.

"What do you do in your free time?"

"I don't have much of it, but I like to tinker with my motorcycle."

"So you don't just sit around with your feet up and have people wait on you?"

Bob started laughing, "No, no. I see where you're going."

"Okay, so we've established you are not lazy, so let's talk about the real reasons you struggle with exercising regularly."

In situations like Bob's, the reason he doesn't exercise may be related to some combination of not enjoying it, lacking time, not knowing what to do, not having a past history of exercising, or not seeing the benefits. Labeling himself "lazy" is inaccurate and does nothing to solve the problem.

Likewise, labeling someone a "jerk" does nothing to define problems with the relationship. Therefore, the relationship probably won't improve. Saying you failed a test because you're *stupid* prevents you from looking at the real reason you didn't perform well.

In most instances, *labeling* is a poor way of explaining our behavior. We are unintentionally reasoning our way out of a solution. In other situations, using labels can be a copout. When you label yourself stupid, lazy, disorganized, or lacking willpower, you're saying you can't change—and that lets you off the hook for managing your weight. Labeling other people as jerks means you can't fix the relationship, so why bother trying?

Emotional Reasoning

Most of the thought patterns we've looked at in this chapter are based on emotional reasoning. This type of reasoning occurs when we think or feel something so strongly that we believe it must be true. In other words—we're fooling ourselves.

Emotional reasoning can stem from positive or negative emotions. Imagine an engaged couple who can't keep their hands off each other. We'll call them Jack and Susie. Everything about their communication with each other indicates they're madly in love. Although he wouldn't admit it to his friends, Jack has learned to like chick flicks because Susie loves to snuggle up close to him and watch them. Susie's phone is full of cute selfies of the two of them just hanging out. One day you get a chance to talk to the couple.

"I'm just curious. The two of you are obviously in love, but every couple has problems. Susie, can you tell me one thing about Jack that sort of gets on your nerves?"

Susie looks at you and then back at Jack and sort of giggles while brushing the side of his cheek with the back side of her slightly bent index finger. With a glimmer in her eyes she says, "Really, there're nothing about Jack I don't absolutely love. He is my everything; we're soulmates."

You try to keep a straight face as Jack gently leans forward and kisses Susie on the forehead. Then you ask Jack the same question. "How about you, Jack? There must be something about Susie that sort of bothers you."

Jack responds, "I guess nobody is perfect, but I think Susie is perfect for me. I mean look at her, she is absolutely beautiful and she treats me like a king."

This interaction is an example of being *blinded by love*, which in short is emotional reasoning. These powerful feelings influence their reasoning. Let's fast-forward five years. Susie and Jack are now in marital therapy because things have turned sour in their relationship. Jack sits at the end of the sofa and Susie is as far away from him as the furniture will allow. Their bodies lean away from each other and their eyes no longer sparkle. In fact, Susie's eyes seem to squint with anger and Jack's are constantly rolling into the back of his head as Susie unleashes her laundry list of complaints. The therapist asks Susie a simple question.

"Tell me what attracted you to Jack, why you fell in love with him in the first place."

With her arms folded she sighs, and says, "Honestly, I can't tell you. I don't know if we were truly ever in love. We have just really never connected like some couples."

The therapist poses the same question to Jack. "What about you, Jack? Why did you fall in love with Susie?"

"That's a hard question. We were working at the same company and neither of us was in a relationship. Maybe we got together because it was convenient."

Let's compare the two conversations with the couple. Before they were married, Jack and Susie were blinded by love. Now they're blinded by anger and negative feelings toward each other. In both situations they weren't thinking rationally because their feelings got in the way. Somewhere in between these two extremes lies a happy medium for Jack and Susie. Perhaps the therapist can help them reach that point.

Emotional reasoning permeates many areas of our lives, including relationships, career, self-image, and certainly weight management. Having a strong emotional reaction each time you see the scale move in the wrong direction may cause a surge of negative emotions that leads to irrational thinking. Maybe you vow to eat nothing all day forgetting that each time you try this it ends in disaster. Or perhaps you *feel* strongly that you'll never succeed and, as a result, you stop trying to eat right or stay active.

Demands

The psychologist Albert Ellis is famous for telling people to "stop shoulding on yourself." I can't think of an area in life where the word "should" is used more often than with diet, exercise and weight management.

- I should get up early in the morning to work out.
- I should take my lunch to work.
- I guess I should join the gym again.
- I know I shouldn't eat so much ice cream.
- We should get back to shopping from a grocery list.
- I should just tell my husband not to buy me chocolate.

Why do we use this word? In some situations the word *should* may bring good results by reminding us of things that are *right* and most consistent with our beliefs. *I should study for my test instead of going out with my friends.* Once you say this you know you'll feel guilty if you go out. Since you don't like feeling guilty, you stay home even though you don't want to. Doing well on the test reinforces your strategy to use the word *should*.

But sometimes, *should* is a way we superficially deal with a situation to make us feel a little bit better. If I am talking to my dentist and say, "I know I should floss more often," this statement probably won't lead to action. It's used to relieve the embarrassment I feel for all the problems with my teeth. This type of *should* makes me feel like I'm doing something, even when I'm not and have no intention to. In a situation like this, using *should* takes the pressure off, but may actually make it less likely that I'll change my behavior.

If you want to manage your weight long-term, *shoulding* yourself is not the best strategy. As in the dentist example above, it may actually prevent us from doing what's important. Even if you have short-term success guilting yourself into action, this won't be effective in the long run. Even if it worked, who wants to feel guilty or pressured all the time? Telling yourself you have to do something strips away your perception of freedom and can lead to feeling disgruntled and even angry.

Imagine if the Christmas-time bell ringer for the Salvation Army stopped you at the grocery store, shook his finger at you, and said, "I know you have enough money to contribute to help us. You should stop thinking so much about *yourself* and *your* family and give to those who barely have enough to eat or don't have a home to live in."

> *Telling yourself you have to do something strips away your perception of freedom and can lead to feeling disgruntled and even angry.*

How would you respond? I suspect you'd react in one of two ways: Either you'd walk on by (even if you were considering a donation before he started his diatribe), or you'd feel guilty enough to reluctantly throw some cash into the red container. No matter what you decided to do, you wouldn't feel good about the bell ringer—and next time you'd probably use a different entrance to avoid the red kettle.

No one likes being strong-armed, so why do it to yourself? Telling yourself you *should* eat and exercise in a certain way will make those activities less desirable. You're almost certain to (1) rebel against yourself, or (2) engage in exercise and dieting with a chip on your shoulder. Either way, you won't be able to keep this going very long.

In a way, you're telling yourself you aren't smart enough, good enough, or disciplined enough to make choices based on what you truly want.

If I tell myself, "I should have an apple, not the cake," I end up losing no matter which food I choose. If I eat the apple I feel deprived. If I eat the cake I feel guilty. If I eat both of them I feel even worse.

Maybe you substitute a different word for *should*:

I have to

I need to

I ought to

I'm supposed to

These phrases yield the same results. If we want to make lasting behavior changes and feel good about it, we need to stop talking to ourselves that way. Be nice to yourself. A simple change in words can make all the difference. Instead of using those demanding *should* words, try something like this:

I could have the apple or I could have the cake.

I could go to the gym or I could stay home.

I can take the elevator or walk up the stairs.

I could order dessert or wait until later.

You are giving yourself a choice—not a command. With this approach you can weigh the options, looking at the pros, cons, and consequence of each decision. Sometimes you might decide on the cake, but you needn't feel guilty if you figured out how it could work within your larger goal of being healthy. If you decide on the apple you don't need to feel deprived, because you decided it was the best decision.

As you go through the day, watch for the times you "should" yourself and try viewing these situations as a choice.

Taking the Blame

Are you one of those people who take the blame for almost everything bad that happens around you? If your kid makes bad decisions, it's your fault. If your boss is curt with you, you must have done something wrong. If you get sick, God is punishing you for some indiscretion. If the cashier is rude when you ask her a question, you must be more clueless than all the other shoppers. Being able to see our faults is an honorable and psychologically healthy attribute. Blaming ourselves for everything bad that happens is not.

I often ask groups of overweight people what causes obesity. I'm always curious to hear their answers, especially in a group where the facilitator (me) isn't obese. The different responses often clue me in to which of them are self-blamers. Even the kindest people who would never cast undue blame on someone else, often unfairly blame themselves. Here's what I often hear from these folks:

"This probably doesn't apply to everyone, but for me it's all about my lack of lack self-control."

"I follow a see-food diet, when I see it I eat it" (self-deprecating humor).

"I use food for comfort."

"I'm just lazy" (a self-blaming label).

"It's my lack of motivation."

I find it interesting that people who tend to blame themselves rarely mention genetics or even the environment as contributing factors. Does the self-criticism help with weight management? Some of my patients lie awake at night reviewing everything they ate that day; blaming themselves for being weak. This doesn't help them eat better the next day— it just makes them feel miserable and guilty. When it comes to understanding the reasons for obesity, the psychological sweet spot includes taking some personal responsibility, but also remembering the things we can't change, such as genetics and some environmental factors. When you cut back on self-blaming, it clears the way for creative problem solving. The focus becomes less personal and more practical. You are more likely to succeed and feel good about your accomplishments.

> *When you cut back on self-blaming, it clears the way for creative problem solving.*

Rationalization: It's Not My Fault

Another fallacy of thought is the opposite of the *taking the blame* concept we just covered. Instead of blaming themselves for everything, some people blame others or their situation in life. From these folks, I hear such statements as:

"My parents were overweight, so I inherited this problem."

"I have a slow metabolism."

"We were forced to eat everything on our plates when I was a kid."

"Nobody in my family will eat the healthy foods I cook."

"I can't afford a gym membership and healthy food costs too much."

Sometimes we come up with complicated explanations for our behavior so we don't have to take responsibility for it. Yes, we do live in a culture that promotes weight gain and inactivity, but we still have choices. Some rationalizers are the defensive, angry types and others are intellectuals, debating like high paid defense attorneys. Some of us have spent years "spinning" the responsibility of our actions to make it someone else's fault when we can't reach our goals. Always shifting the blame bogs down our ability to achieve health goals.

I met with Betty regularly for over a year. She wanted a reasonable diet plan and, like many of my clients, had already tried many diets. Like others, she lost weight and regained it many times. Betty came to our center because she felt the other plans were the wrong plans; they weren't realistic and weren't prescribed by professionals. Although she tried some fad diets, some of the programs she attempted to follow were healthy and reasonable.

One thing I hoped to accomplish with Betty was to figure out why she had a difficult time sustaining the plans. But Betty wasn't interested in that approach. The longer I worked with her, the more evident it became that Betty struggled with rationalization and blaming. She fell off the program for the weekend because of what someone said on Friday afternoon at work. Her parents taught her to eat emotionally. She didn't exercise because of sore knees and limited income for a gym membership. Any suggestion I made led to a, "Yeah, but that won't work for me because," response.

Even open-ended questions such as, "What would you like to get out of today's session?" led to extended stories of how others were responsible for her problems. Clearly, Betty had a communication style full of avoidance. She avoided taking responsibility because she believed she wasn't emotionally strong enough to handle it. I learned she also suffered from depression, and in the past, admitting her imperfections and mistakes caused her mood to spiral downward. She found it easier—and mentally safer—to keep looking for a better diet plan, a different therapist, or more supportive friends.

I wish every patient interaction I describe was a success, but Betty's wasn't, at least not during the time we worked together. When we attempted to address some of the underlying thought processes that could be helpful in the long run, Betty discontinued treatment.

As with Betty's case, thoughts are the seeds of our beliefs and attitudes. They influence our emotional reactions and ultimately our behavior. Once we understand the type of thinking that makes weight management difficult, we can take specific steps to alter our thinking. In the next chapter you'll learn practical strategies to restructure your thoughts and transform your approach to weight management.

Chapter 10

Change Your Mind

LET'S TAKE A quick look at what we've discussed so far:

- Thoughts, emotions, and behavior influence each other—usually behind the scenes where we don't recognize what's happening.

- Many types of destructive thought patterns (fallacies of thought) directly affect our weight management behavior. These harmful and often untrue thoughts turn into beliefs that become part of our identities. We don't even think to question them.

I hope you agree that it's a good idea to change thoughts and beliefs that stand between us and weight management. But how can we do it?

The first thing to remember is that thinking is automated. If we do nothing, we continue to think and behave the same way. Changing our thoughts requires practice and persistence. Earlier you read about the ABCs—activating events that lead to beliefs, followed by a consequence, such as an emotion.

> *One way to practice changing thoughts is to add a **D** to our ABCs. The D stands for **dispute**.*

One way to practice changing thoughts is to add a *D* to our ABCs. The D stands for *dispute*. What are we disputing? We are disputing beliefs that lead to undesirable reactions to situations. Here's an example:

Activating Event:

Joanie vowed to begin eating better, but a co-worker brought her wonderful lemon bars to work on Friday. Joanie ate four of them.

Belief:

I totally blew it today—I have absolutely no self-control! Since today was a disaster, it doesn't really matter what we eat for dinner. We might as well order a pizza with extra cheese tonight—and go ahead and add those dessert bread stick thingies too. I can always get back on track at the beginning of next week.

Consequence: Frustrated with herself for not handling the lemon bar situation well, Joanie feels hopeless about managing day-to-day food choices. She loses focus on her goals and overeats for the rest of the weekend.

Dispute:

Let's look at Joanie's dysfunctional beliefs and how we can dispute them. Thinking she'd already *blown it* for the day and had *absolutely no* self-control are perfect examples of all-or-nothing thoughts that have a tone of failure and hopelessness. The idea that she should go ahead and eat more because she ate too much earlier is emotional reasoning. After having her wallet stolen, would Joanie withdraw money from the bank and set the money on fire? If she accidentally dropped a glass and it broke on her kitchen floor, would she break more dishes, because ten broken glasses are the same as one? When a patient describes it-doesn't-matter feelings, I'm often reminded of the lyrics from my favorite Kenny Wayne Shepherd song. It's like:

...blue on black, tears on a river, push on a shove, it don't mean much... whisper on a scream—doesn't change a thing.

That's how we feel when emotions run high. But feelings are not reality. The extra calories we eat after a snacking mishap aren't the same as a whisper on a scream. They matter. More importantly, these beliefs interfere with your ability to handle slips. Thinking this way ultimately continues the diet-relapse cycle. Just as setting money on fire after getting your wallet stolen is illogical, so is continuing to make poor food choices just because you made one poor choice.

The belief *I can always get back on track at the beginning of next week* is a classic procrastination strategy that gives Joanie permission to think and act irrationally because she'll start fresh at some time in the future. The procrastination thought helps her feel a little better because she has an obscure plan to get back on track. Procrastinating gives Joanie a little psychological space to forget about messing up earlier, so she can eat the pizza and dessert breadsticks without overwhelming guilt. But if Joanie took time to think rationally about her situation, she'd realize that going off the rails for the entire weekend leads to feelings of regret. So how could Joanie think about the lemon bar incident? Consider these ideas:

Disputing "I've already blown it for the today."

Although I'm not happy about eating the lemon bars, I haven't ruined my day. That extra 600 calories is a minor contributor to my weight, especially if I eat reasonably the rest of the evening.

Disputing "I have absolutely no self-control."

That's not true. I have a lot of self-control in many areas of my life. I often refuse buying things to stay within our budget. I don't tell people off every time I have a negative thought about them, and when it comes to food, I've been making good choices more than not-so-good ones for weeks.

Disputing "It doesn't matter what I eat for dinner, we might as well order a pizza."

In actuality what I eat the rest of the evening does matter; it only feels like it doesn't. Making better choices the rest of the day will help me recover from slips more easily in the future. Possibly, Joanie really wants the pizza and dessert breadsticks for dinner. If that is the case, fine, but let that decision arise from rational thoughts that allow her to fully consider the pros and cons. The pizza meal should be her conscious choice, not an emotional reaction.

Disputing "I can always get back on track at the beginning of next week."

Hold on, that isn't a recovery plan—it's a sneaky way of giving myself permission to stay on a path I'll regret later. What can I do right now to get back on track? I'll take a five-minute walk and think about the best way to handle food choices for the rest of the day.

> *The last part of the ABCs (and now D), is to add E.*
>
> *E reminds us to evaluate.*

The last part of the ABCs (and now D), is to add *E*. E reminds us to *evaluate*. At this stage, we examine how facing dysfunctional beliefs about weight management will change our emotions, and then alter our behavior in a positive way.

Did thinking differently about a situation help calm your feelings?

Did you behave in a different way, with less drama and a better outcome?

If you've already begun reacting to situations in a more sensible, thoughtful way, then the thought changing exercises are working. If not, don't feel discouraged. Take time to examine which thoughts are still holding you back. Remember that emotions are not a switch we turn on and off. Even if we begin thinking differently, our emotions can linger awhile. Just because you recognize something isn't true doesn't mean you immediately stop reacting emotionally to the initial thought. Combining the thought restructuring exercises above with deep breathing or moderate exercise may help settle your emotions.

Be Your Own Best Friend

Some people find it difficult to dispute their own thoughts. If you've spent years believing something and feeling a certain way about it, changing your viewpoint is tough. These may be things you learned in childhood and never questioned.

Several strategies can help adjust your perspective. One of the most effective ways to deal with stinkin' thinkin' is asking, "What would I tell a close friend who has dysfunctional thoughts about this exact situation?"

Imagine your friend, a single mom, calls you and says, with a note of hysteria in her voice: "I just got laid off at work. I won't be able to feed my kids. We'll be homeless and my kids will never forgive me for putting them through this. I'm such a loser! If I'd finished college, I'd have a better job and none of this would be happening."

With those thoughts, no wonder she's upset. As a good friend you would be a voice of reason, helping her calm down and see things differently so she can begin problem solving. After expressing your sympathy, you might start by asking if she has any savings or family members who can help. You might have suggestions for finding another job right away. Plus, what evidence does she have that her kids will be traumatized? You might gently point out that the kids are influenced by her reactions. You would certainly remind her that she isn't a loser—hasn't she always provided for her children and found a way when times were tough? In short, you would show your friend a different perspective, talking her down with a combination of affection, calmness, and logic.

Your friend's emotional reaction to losing her job probably stems from thoughts and beliefs about herself, such as: "I'm a failure. I can't control what happens to me and I can't deal with challenges." You would never say those things to her, but she says them to herself.

Have you noticed we sometimes show kindness to our friends while being cruel to ourselves? You wouldn't tell a friend, "Yes, you're a big loser for not finishing school and losing your job. You're going to be homeless and get what you deserve."

Hopefully, you also wouldn't give your friend superficial feedback, like "Stop worrying. Things will work out for the best." Instead, you would dig into her concerns to help her balance logic and emotion so she could stop worrying so much and find a solution to her solvable problems.

When you're trying to dispute your thoughts and beliefs, I challenge you do so as if you were speaking to your best friend. Acknowledge negative thoughts, but also look for a functional perspective that will help you calm your nerves and feel hopeful. See yourself as your own best friend. Disarm negative thoughts and beliefs about yourself by providing facts to the contrary. Accept your imperfections, speak to yourself respectfully, and lift yourself up as you work on making better decisions in the future.

> *I challenge you to see yourself as your own best friend.*

Challenging Our Core Beliefs

The lemon bar and job loss examples illustrate how our thoughts can impact our immediate emotional reactions to situations. Challenging our thoughts as we would when we talk to a close friend goes a long way toward helping us better manage life and our weight. But some of us have entrenched beliefs that influence our perspectives on many life situations. We may be sensitive to certain conditions that trigger these beliefs. Such thoughts and assumptions are typically about others, ourselves, or the world around us. I've alluded to some of these global beliefs throughout the last several chapters. They may include such ideas as:

- People only care about themselves.

- I have to please everyone all of the time or I'm inadequate.

- When people make mistakes they always deserve to be punished.

- Those who care about me won't ever mistreat me.

The difficult part of each of the above examples is that they're partly true. People can be selfish, but that doesn't mean they only care about themselves. It's also admirable to try to help others and get along with them, but this isn't always possible. Justice is something we long for, but what about mercy and forgiveness? And isn't it true that sometimes we can be unkind to those we love? When we hold tightly to the rigid beliefs above, there's little room to forgive others or accept their help. We hold grudges or perhaps feel lonely as we drown in a sea of self-blame. We are highly sensitive to other people's selfishness and easily dismiss their acts of kindness. We demand justice and feel perpetually frustrated when our demands aren't met. We can become people pleasers and expect the same from others.

So how do we handle these or other entrenched core beliefs that cause us distress and impact our physical activity or eating habits? As discussed above, I encourage you to have an internal dialogue with yourself. Be respectful, as though you're discussing an issue with a friend. Also be direct and include facts rather than feelings. What is the evidence that people only care about themselves? What evidence refutes this belief? How about the idea that people who care about you won't ever mistreat you? Have you talked to any couples who've been married a long time? Have you interviewed people who have great relationships with their adult kids? They would most certainly tell you they have mistreated, or been mistreated, at times by the people they love most. Isn't there a place for grace and mercy just as there's a place for working hard to earn something and suffering the consequences when we mess up?

> *Changing core beliefs ever so slightly can make a huge difference in how we respond to situations.*

Tackling these emotion-provoking core beliefs can be a challenge. At some point you accepted them as true. But with work, we can change false assumptions and the cascade of thoughts and behavior that emanates from them.

The good news is—altering core beliefs ever so slightly can make a huge difference in how we respond to situations. After some thought and internal conversation, you may come up with alternative core beliefs. The following perspectives are more reality-based and may help you deal with stressful events:

- Most people care about others but still act selfishly at times.

- I want to make others happy, but in the end, happiness is a choice.

- Everyone makes mistakes. The timing and severity of consequences aren't always up to me.

- I won't be anyone's doormat, but even people who care deeply about me will occasionally be insensitive to my needs.

Working on your own, you can come up with alternative beliefs the same way we challenged thoughts about eating lemon bars and being laid off.

First, examine an activating event (A) that triggered deep-seated beliefs (B) and your emotions and behavior (C). Perhaps you realize you need to dispute certain core beliefs (D) and make adjustments. Because these beliefs are global and affect large areas of your life, think of them as personal mission statements or proverbs. Continue to evaluate (E) the wisdom of these beliefs as you apply them to hardships and life transitions.

Write It Down

As you work on changing your thoughts and "friending" yourself, creating a Thought Log with the ABCDE format will help you analyze events in your life and track progress. You might dedicate a special journal just for this exercise.

1. When something upsets you, jot down the activating event (A), dysfunctional beliefs (B) and emotional consequences (C) of your thoughts.

2. Consider what thinking category causes you to feel bad (all or nothing thinking, emotional reasoning, etc.).

3. Now you can dispute (D) the thought and replace it with a kinder, factual, probable, and useful perspective.

4. Finally, you can evaluate (E) how strongly you felt the initial emotion. Perhaps in the beginning you felt frustrated at an intensity of 90 on a scale of 1 to 100.

5. Record the new rating of frustration (1 to 100) after you begin thinking differently.

You may not like keeping a journal with this much structure, and that's okay. But I do recommend you take time to evaluate how the information in this chapter and Chapter 9 affects your life.

Sit down with paper and pen, or at your computer, and write about which fallacies of thought have kept you from losing weight and sustaining that weight loss. You don't need to write a novel. Don't worry about spelling or grammar and feel free to use bullet points instead of sentences.

I suggest you start with writing how the environment and your thinking influenced you to regain weight in the past. Suppose you gained weight after a combination of events— you hurt your foot in October, followed by the stress and social events of the holidays, and then you felt discouraged and gave up. What if you changed your interpretation of those events—your thoughts and beliefs? Would the story have a different ending?

Write about how you could have changed the environment to ensure better success. Then try writing how you could change your thoughts if you couldn't change the environment. How could this situation end with a better outcome? While you're at it, write about several of those possible good outcomes. This will show you how changing your thoughts could lead to much better results.

This writing exercise will be like a dress rehearsal for similar challenges in the future. Instead of falling into the same traps as before, you've prepared yourself to respond in a healthier way. As with anything you practice the right way, you'll soon develop thinking skills and new confidence to overcome future challenges to maintaining a healthy weight.

Chapter 11

Good Goals — With or Without Clothes

PEOPLE I COUNSEL are usually seeing me because they haven't been able to achieve their goals for weight and health. Many of them are successful in other areas of their lives. At work, they create objectives, manage budgets, and delegate work to get results. Goal setting is easy for them in their roles as teachers, accountants, and sales associates. Even those who aren't paid for their work, such as the stay-at-home moms and dads, are often amazingly good at organizing their lives when it comes to grocery shopping, getting the kids to and from various events, paying bills, cleaning house, preparing meals, and volunteering for community organizations. I've worked with physicians, nurses, and veterinarians who preserve life when they accomplish their goals, and business owners and executives whose work supports thousands of people.

Many of these folks are efficient, well-oiled machines when it comes to getting things done. They've learned to set realistic short-term and long-term goals and the results are impressive. But when health goals are at stake, it's often a totally different story. The machine becomes clunky in one area of their lives and out of sync in another.

Where do they go wrong? Their intentions are nonspecific, unrealistic, poorly thought out, or rehashed from past unmet goals.

Many of my patients refuse to continue setting nutrition or fitness-related goals. Their attitude is, "Why would I set a goal

I know I won't achieve? Then I'll feel even worse!" They exist between a rock and a hard place, knowing goals are important, but also knowing the pain of failure.

I often ask clients what they'd tell their children, grandkids or other young people about goals. "Would you tell them to forget about goals because you'll only disappoint yourself when you don't achieve them?"

That question usually evokes a blank stare followed by a nervous smile. "No, I *guess* not."

"So what *would* you say?" The responses to this question have several themes:

- Goals are important.
- They help us clarify where we want to go and how we can get there.
- Achieving goals is rewarding in and of itself.
- Not achieving goals can provide lessons on how to set better goals.
- Setting goals can motivate us into action.
- Goals can help us separate essential things from all the rest.

In the early 1980s, George T. Doran, a corporate consultant, coined the acronym *S.M.A.R.T.* for effective goal setting. Since then, educators have adapted the term to meet their needs for different disciplines. I borrowed George's ideas to help clients remember the importance of weight-related goals.

B SMART

This acronym is easy to remember and the letters stand for the following:

B= Behavior (make sure your goals are about behavior, not just outcomes such as weight)

S=Specific (what, when, and where)

M=Measurable (calories, servings of vegetables, miles walked, steps, minutes of exercise, etc.)

A=Achievable (goals are realistic even when unexpected events occur)

R=Reason (why is this important?)

T=Time Frame (what is the length of the goal—one day, a week, a month?)

Let's review each of these points individually and a little out of order.

And The Reason Is?

When we set weight-related goals, they should have meaning and a clear reason for existing. I end most of my sessions with a goal setting exercise by asking the patient to tell me what he or she wants to achieve before our next meeting together. Sometimes people tell me what I want to hear, just to end our session. An attitude of "Let me set these goals so I can get out of here," isn't helpful to either of us. The goal is selected, but it doesn't have meaning.

Neither is it helpful when someone chooses a goal that's important to someone else or because of feeling obligated. You probably won't be successful if you set a goal because a psychologist, doctor, minister, or family member twisted your arm.

Before you set a goal, ask, "Why is this goal important to me?" Write the answer in specific terms. By specific, I mean avoid grand, general statements such as, "I want to be healthy," or "I want to improve my quality of life." Those are not specific reasons to eat better or lose weight, and they don't spur you to action. I once heard a speaker discuss this topic and his technique was so effective that I've been using it for twenty years. Here's an example:

When my patient, Barbara, announced she wanted to set the goal of tracking food in a food journal, I asked, "Why is this important to you?"

"Because tracking my food helps me pay attention to what I'm eating."

"Why is it important for you to pay attention to your eating?"

"Because it helps me lose weight."

"So you can what?"

"So I can be healthier."

"So you can what?"

"So I can live longer and have a better quality of life."

"Live longer for what?"

"To see my grandkids graduate from high school."

"Anything else?"

"I have a lot of things I still want to do."

"Like what?"

"I want to travel to Europe with my husband after I retire and I want to hike the Grand Canyon someday. I want to ride bikes with my youngest grandkids and my future grandkids.

"What else?"

"I just want to feel better."

"Why does that matter to you?"

"Well, I won't have to take as much medicine and I'll have energy to do more things."

"Can you give me more examples?"

"When I feel better, I like to read and learn about new things. I enjoy work more, I laugh more, and my life is extra meaningful. When I feel bad it's all about me. I want to rest; I just barely get through the day. It's easier to enjoy almost everything when I have more energy and less pain."

The point of this exercise is to distill the reasons for our goals into smaller and more specific ideas. These new, small-scale goals are meaningful, and even joyful. In the above example, Barbara's food journal is tied to quality time with her grandkids, enjoying her job, laughing, and hiking the Grand Canyon. When the rubber hits the road, these factors offer greater motivation than simply telling herself that keeping a food journal will help her lose weight and get healthier. Visualizing all the things she wants to do drives her to accomplish her goal.

The *B* Is for Behavior

Outcome goals are king in weight management, but they shouldn't be.

I will lose 30 pounds and keep it off.

I'm going to get off my blood pressure medication.

This year I will run a 10k race.

There's nothing wrong with these goals. Losing weight, getting off medication, and fitness events are all good things. But if this is the extent of goal setting you may fall short. Each outcome goal we set should be coupled with specific actions to support the goal. These actions are called behavioral goals. Although a baseball coach may have a goal to win the championship, nothing is going to happen without specific behavioral goals for the team. Likewise, if your desire to lose 30 pounds isn't coupled with clear-cut behavioral goals, it probably won't happen. Action-oriented goals for weight management can include anything that directly or indirectly impacts weight:

Self-weighing	Food journaling	Weighing/ measuring food
Shopping from a grocery list	Meal planning	Tracking steps
Going to the gym	Walking the dog	Rating hunger/ fullness

Sleep	Time spent watching TV	Alcohol intake
Dining out	Playing in a sports league	Eating less at night
Eating at the table	Walking on lunch hour	Prayer habits
Meditation	Journaling thoughts	Batch cooking
Seeing a therapist	Taking an exercise class	Attending support group

Specific *(S)* and Measurable *(M)*

Setting criteria you can measure is an excellent way to find and define specific goals. People frequently tell me their weight-related goals are to *exercise more this month, eat better,* or *get back on track.* What do these mean? One more step, one more bite of broccoli? Is getting back on track just a frame of mind or an actual set of behaviors?

Suppose you want to focus on increasing vegetables, eating breakfast, and reducing your calorie intake late at night. Specific and measurable goals could be:

- I will eat two cups of vegetables at least four days this week.

- I will eat something before 9:30 a.m. six days this week.

- I will track the calories in my snacks after dinner and stay under 300 for at least five days this week.

If your goal involves physical activity, take a few minutes to think about what you'll do, how often you'll do it, and the amount of time you'll spend. Also consider factors that affect your activities, such as thunderstorms (if it's raining I will walk on the treadmill instead of riding my bike outside). For example:

- This week I will walk outside or on my treadmill before work for at least 30 minutes.
- I will go to Zumba class on Saturday.
- I will wear my Fitbit every day this week and reach 10,000 steps on at least five days.
- I will walk on my lunch hour on Tuesday, Thursday, and Friday.

Generally speaking, the more specific and detailed the plan, the better. On one occasion, however, I got more information than I bargained for. Marie told me her plan was to continue doing resistance training three times per week with rubber tubing. I asked her what days and times she would work out and which exercises she would do. Marie told me she waited until the evening to do her exercises because that's when her husband was home and he liked to watch her workout. Straight faced she added, "He likes it because I work out in the buff." Since the success rates for maintaining marriages and fitness programs aren't so great, I supported this plan. I decided to forego my usual questions about exercise form and technique and assumed she was working all her major muscle groups. Since that day, I always feel the need to wipe down rubber tubing before I use it at the gym!

A = Attainable

This step of goal setting is where things often fall apart. In our minds we know what's recommended, ideal, or possible—and so we set goals accordingly. We ignore that the planets would have to align in perfect order to create the circumstances for us to achieve these goals. If you typically eat three vegetables per month, immediately transitioning to five servings per day is highly improbable. Even though 10,000 steps is recommended, increasing from 4,000 to 6,000 may be more realistic in the beginning. This approach worked well for Janet.

When Janet told me she was wearing her pedometer faithfully, I didn't really believe this was true. I couldn't imagine she was truly walking only 900 to 1,200 steps each day. *She must be only wearing it a few hours during the day; maybe the pedometer is a lemon or the batteries are bad.* The average American, who is notoriously sedentary, accumulates five times as many steps. Although she was overweight, Janet wasn't disabled in any way. Her knees seemed to be in shape to handle walking and she didn't complain of any other limitations. Janet would have to increase her walking by a factor of 10 to reach the recommended 10,000 steps per day.

When she described her lifestyle things began to make sense. She was a busy account manager at her firm but worked from home. She parked at her desk all day, only getting up to go to the bathroom or kitchen, both near her office. When she finished working, she would sometimes run an errand or do some light house cleaning, but that was about it for physical activity. In the evening Janet often returned to her computer to finish work, fall into the abyss of social media, or play solitaire. She and her husband would also watch an hour or two of TV. She'd never been an exerciser but was open to the idea of becoming more physically active. She had recently lost weight without exercise but knew her chances of keeping it off were not good unless she moved more. Janet also wanted to feel better. She felt sluggish. Like a toddler who can't sit still, her body yearned for movement.

She started with a goal of 3,000 steps each day, which she achieved easily just by getting out of her chair more during her work day and doing a daily errand that required some walking. After several weeks of this, we set a goal of 5,000 steps per day at least five days per week. She was able to accomplish this on the weekend by doing yard work and more housecleaning. On work days she decided to walk for 20 minutes when she took a break for lunch. Janet enjoyed the concrete aspect of tracking her steps and the challenge of reaching her goals. She was also motivated by the fact that she felt more energetic, could concentrate better throughout the day, and slept soundly at night.

> *Sometimes our goals yield observable positive results and sometimes they simply keep us from sliding backward.*

The next goal was to reach 8,000 steps at least three days per week. Again, the weekends were easier. Janet added a 40-minute walk to her already established weekend routine. She also began taking a 40-minute walk with her husband on Wednesday or Thursday evenings. Janet and I continued to set progressive goals and after six months she took 7,000 to 11,000 steps at least five days per week. We didn't quite reach 10,000 steps every day, but we were close. Janet was now walking in place during long conference calls and enthusiastically signed up for her first 5K. She was always excited to tell me about her new step record, which finally hit 15,000 per day, thanks to a 40-minute Saturday walk plus a trip to the flea market.

Setting attainable goals requires setting aside our *should* thoughts and *all or nothing thinking* and focusing on progress, not perfection. Goals need not be like a light switch we flip on and off, going full force and then regressing back to nothing. Instead our goals can be more like a dimmer switch that's always turned on, sometimes shining brightly and at other times softly illuminating. No matter the intensity of our goals, the act of setting them helps keep us mindful of long-term objectives. Each month, week, or day, consider what you can realistically accomplish. During a busy week of travel you may focus on maintaining your weight by getting to the hotel gym three times and avoiding dessert and alcohol when dining out in the evening. When you're at home with better control of the environment, you can turn the dimmer switch up to more frequent exercise, lower-calorie food preparation, and a greater variety of vegetables than were available while traveling. The famed Scottish novelist Robert Louis Stevenson put it this way: "Don't judge each day by the harvest you reap but by the seeds that you plant."

"T" Is for Time Frame

Short-term and long-term goals are both important, especially when we focus on losing a substantial amount of weight. Losing 30 pounds means you have to create a 105,000 calorie deficit over an extended period of time. Unfortunately, once you lose weight, the hardest part of weight management awaits you—maintenance. To keep the weight off you'll need to sustain most of the behavior that helped you lose weight in the first place. A 30-pound weight loss from conventional treatments may take six months to a year as you consistently burn more calories than you consume. Therefore, you'll need to set many short-term goals along the way. You will have to *manage* your weight, just as supervisors manage a business, frequently evaluating success and failure while readjusting your goals and objectives.

A common error in goal setting is to have long-term goals without setting enough goals for the short run. In some circumstances I discourage long-term goals, such as overall weight loss, until a client has a chance to set short-term behavioral goals and see how much work weight loss requires. A *healthy weight* is the weight you reach when you do healthy things over an extended period of time. This can't be determined by a chart, a formula, or even the weight you felt great at 20 years ago. You're setting yourself up for disappointment if you set a weight goal you can only reach if you behave in a way that isn't healthy or realistic to sustain.

That's why specific, shorter-term goals with a wait-and-see approach are often more effective. You'll get immediate returns by feeling better and becoming more fit, instead of holding onto a distant "pie in the sky" goal. The idea of that goal may still exist, but it won't be your main focus.

Although no secret formula exists for timing your goals and reviewing progress, I encourage at least weekly goal-setting sessions during the early stages of weight loss. Once a week you can either meet with a professional, a peer, or yourself to review how you did with the previous week's goals. If you achieved them, how did you do it? If you didn't, why not? Were your goals unrealistic, not specific enough, or maybe not that important to you? Or was it a problem with execution? Do you need a more specific action plan, such as making sure you go to the grocery store over the weekend and stock up on food to cook healthier meals? Perhaps your goal of exercising in the morning will only work if you have a plan that helps you get to bed earlier the night before. Did you put everyone else's needs in front of your own? You might reevaluate your thinking.

Over time, accomplishing these short-term goals may lead to habits you follow without thinking. When this happens, weight management becomes easier. However, because obesity is a chronic, relapsing condition, I encourage you to be diligent about frequently evaluating your progress. If your behavior starts to drift in the wrong direction, you can quickly identify the problem areas and use goal setting to help you get back on track. This may be as simple as weighing daily and observing your weight graph once a month to spot trends. Some of my long-term clients, even if they're doing well, return to the office every month or two for exactly this reason.

> *Because obesity is a chronic, relapsing condition, I encourage you to be diligent about frequently evaluating your progress.*

Chapter 12

Relapse Prevention

"HI, DAN, HOW are you today?"

Dan walked toward me with his arthritic limp, grinned, and held out his hand. "Better than I was," he answered predictably, "but not quite where I wanna be."

Dan was a client I always looked forward to seeing. A witty 46-year old, he owned a flooring business in a nearby town. He'd managed to finish college after a childhood of poverty, worked hard, and built his business from the ground up. He often smiled as he talked about his loyal employees, many of whom had stayed with him since the business opened 15 years earlier. When he talked about his family, Dan's eyes would soften and shine. "My wife is the greatest woman in the world. My daughter's getting married in the fall and my son will graduate with his engineering degree next spring."

Dan was living a life that far exceeded his childhood dreams. Though not wealthy by Wall Street standards, in his mind he was the richest man in the world. However, while living the American dream Dan had ignored his health to focus on business and family. Although his doctor advised him to make lifestyle changes, Dan didn't follow that advice. His wife worried about his weight, bad knees, and rising blood pressure. He responded to her concerns with his usual you-only-live-once, happy-go-lucky attitude and continued his unhealthy patterns.

Dan's eating habits were to blame for his worsening health. He often bought lunch for his entire office staff and would eat whatever they ordered on any given day. Although his wife was willing to cook, Dan enjoyed taking her out to eat. He spent most evenings winding down with one or two rum and cokes and a salty snack or two. This lifestyle led to a steady weight gain over ten years.

An eye-opening experience led Dan to seek treatment at our center. One morning after a restless night of sleep, he decided to check his weight. Maybe the seeds planted by his wife or doctor had started to germinate, or perhaps for some reason he noticed the dusty scale tucked away in the bathroom closet. He dragged the old analog scale out from behind a box of cleaning supplies, set the scale on his tiled floor, and stepped on the black rubber surface. The red dial quickly snapped to the 300-pound maximum and vibrated slightly as it tried to go beyond its limits.

Dan was shocked. He had no idea he weighed that much. "This is really bad," he muttered. "I can't even weigh myself on a normal bathroom scale." All day he thought about his weight, his blood pressure, and the difficulty he had playing a round of golf, and the sleep apnea that left him feeling drowsy throughout the day, even occasionally dozing off at his desk during work. And he had pain. A once-in-awhile ibuprofen pill had become a regular medication to help him walk during the day and control the knee pain that awakened him in the middle of the night.

Dan's wake-up call came from seeing that red dial max out on his bathroom scales. He realized if he didn't stop this weight trajectory, he wouldn't be able to live the way he wanted — and he had a lot to live for.

Dan's motivation translated into action. Every two weeks he came to my office, down another four or five pounds. Occasionally Sheila, his office manager, called to tell me Dan was running five or ten minutes late, but he never missed.

After five months of treatment, Dan had lost 60 pounds. He was playing more golf, helping prepare dinners at home, and his office staff had shaped up too, keeping the refrigerator stocked with fruit, raw veggies, and low-fat dip to accompany the sandwiches they ordered for lunch. Dan told me Sheila and one of his salesmen had lost over 20 pounds each since he started the program.

Even though he'd found his groove for weight loss, Dan wanted to keep meeting with me every other week because it kept him accountable. We discussed that at some point in time things would get harder and he accepted this as a challenge.

Then one day Dan didn't show up for his usual Tuesday afternoon appointment; Sheila didn't call either. Somewhat concerned about his out-of-character absence, I called his personal phone and office phone, but nobody answered, so I left messages. No one returned my call. A week went by and I called his home phone and again had to leave a message. A month had passed and I had thought a lot about Dan. "Why did he stop treatment?" Although I don't make a habit of harassing patients who no longer want to remain in treatment, Dan wasn't a typical patient and his absence didn't make sense. "I'll try one last time," I thought. Like before, six rings and voice mail. Three weeks passed and finally I got a return call.

"Hello Dave, this is Suzanne Smith. My husband Dan Smith was one of your patients at the weight loss center."

"Of course, Suzanne, thank you for calling me."

"You left a couple of messages for Dan and he wanted me to call you. He would talk to you himself, but he's very sick and weak. A few days after you last met with him he started to have abdominal pain and nausea that wouldn't go away. He went to his doctor and at first they thought it was his gallbladder. Then they ran some other tests and found out he had pancreatic cancer." She spoke in a matter-of-fact, well-rehearsed tone.

My throat tightened. "Oh, no, I am so sorry, Suzanne."

Her voice softened as she explained his prognosis. "The cancer is progressing fast and there isn't much we can do other than try to keep him comfortable. We wanted to thank you for your help; Dan felt so good until his symptoms came on all of a sudden."

"I can only imagine everything that's going on for you guys right now, and your call means a lot to me. Please tell Dan hello for me." I hung up the phone and stared at my office wall.

The news shattered my expectations. Dan worked so hard to change his lifestyle—and what was his reward? The things we both believed would prolong his life probably wouldn't give him a single extra second on this earth. Everything he worked for was taken away without warning. I wondered if he had regrets. If Dan had known he'd become so ill, would he have tried to lose weight? About three weeks after my conversation with his wife, Dan died.

I decided to attend his wake with the plan of quietly signing the registry, introducing myself to his wife, and then leaving. I wanted to pay my respects, and to be honest, I needed to find closure to my relationship with him. I arrived at the funeral home to find the parking lot overflowing with cars and a mass of people gathered outside. I quickly realized what I learned about Dan in a clinical setting only scratched the surface of who he was and the impact he made on people in his community. The visitation line stretched from the front to the back of the seating area and then twisted back and forth in the foyer like an amusement park line. The length of the line told me it would be hours before I reached the front to pay my respects. On another night I might have been able to wait, but that night I needed to lead a bariatric support group.

Even though I wouldn't be able to see Dan or his family members, I wanted to stay as long as possible. So I stood in the back of the barely moving line, far from the seriousness of what was taking place at the front of the funeral home. No one was crying, hugging, or being introduced to family members. I couldn't hear anyone saying "I'm so sorry" or "if you need anything, please let me know." At the back of the line I was in a space somewhat removed from the emotion, stuffed into the foyer with seventy or eighty other people. I saw middle-aged people with their young adult children waiting in line. These were probably families who knew Dan through his kids. I spotted a few fidgety men wearing khakis and three-button shirts who seemed to be talking about sports or something more superficial than the event of the evening. "Golfing buddies," I told myself.

I listened to the conversation from a small group of Dan's close friends in front of me. They had seen him regularly over the past year and began discussing his intentional weight loss as well as the weight loss he suffered from cancer.

"He looked and felt so good before he got sick," one man said.

"Yeah, I'd never seen him that trim," another responded before changing the subject.

After hearing those brief comments, I felt a sense of accomplishment. Even though our time together was short, I had a part in helping Dan feel better and achieve something important to him. Dan was not on a miserable diet, denying himself everything he wanted. He didn't isolate himself from others to eat special food or to spend hours at a gym. In fact it was quite the opposite. Dan unintentionally became a health advocate, a leader of sorts. People saw what he had and they wanted it, too.

Dan's death reminded me that our time on this planet isn't guaranteed and can be cut short for no apparent reason. As a result, I became less interested in helping people follow pitifully unpleasant diets. I focused more on encouraging people to find a peaceful balance in their journey to a healthier weight.

Purposeful living often means finding joy in self-denial. The daily satisfaction we feel when overcoming challenges, caring for ourselves, and knowing we're an inspiration to others far outweighs the feelings we get from feeding our immediate desires. Although Dan didn't reap all the long-term benefits of losing weight and living a longer life, the short-term effects of his efforts were just as meaningful. He lived life fully until he became sick and his weight loss was part of a broader personal transformation that made an impact on others, even me.

I began to wonder what would have happened with Dan if the cancer cells hadn't invaded his body. Could he have kept the weight off? Or, like most others, would he have succumbed to the neurochemical, metabolic, psychological, and environmental influences that contribute to weight regain? Would those weight-gain promoting factors have been as powerful and persistent as his unstoppable cancer cells?

Even though statistics tell me Dan would probably have regained his weight, he seemed to have a perspective that could defy the odds and prevent a relapse into old patterns. My time with Dan led me to think a great deal about who succeeds long-term with weight management efforts. I began considering relapse prevention early in my work with other clients, focusing on behavior and perspectives they could sustain long-term.

Batter Up

Weight management is unlike many disciplines in the medical field. When a surgeon operates to remove a gallbladder, the operation is almost always successful. When you take an antibiotic for an infection you usually get better. When you wear a cast, the bone generally heals. Weight management is more like baseball than medicine. If you're a good major league hitting coach, your players may get a base hit three out of ten times. Your hitters may only hit a home run once every 20-30 at bats. Like hitting a 90-mile per hour fastball, weight management is hard. The National Health and Nutrition Examination Survey (NHANES) is a program of studies that includes ongoing assessment of weight. One study from data including over 14,000 people sheds light on how difficult weight management can be.

The figure below shows the percentages of people able to lose weight and keep it off for at least one year. As you can see, losing and keeping off 5% of weight (a 12-pound weight loss if you weigh 240 pounds) happens for just over one-third of people. This is sort of like hitting singles. The probability of losing and keeping off 20% of your body weight (48 pounds if you weigh 240 pounds) is similar to the average professional baseball player's chances of hitting a homerun at any given at bat—4.4% or 1 out of 23.

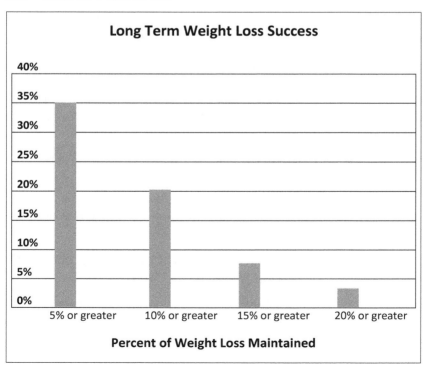

One big problem with weight management is that most of us want to hit a home run; we forget that singles matter. Additional research tells us that a 5 to 10% weight loss improves health, helps prevent diseases like type 2 diabetes, and improves other health conditions such as high blood pressure.

It's important to point out that the NHANES data don't differentiate between people who had bariatric surgery and those who lost weight without it. However, during the time of the study only about one out of every 2500 people had bariatric surgery, suggesting almost all these data relate to people who chose not to have surgery.

Weight loss after bariatric surgery is much greater than this, but those patients also risk short and long-term complications. In addition, most bariatric surgery procedures aren't appropriate for people who have less than 75 pounds of excess weight (gastric banding procedures are exceptions and can be performed for people with various medical conditions who are 30 to 40 pounds or more overweight).

The following section on relapse prevention isn't about hitting home runs or being happy with singles. Instead, I want to explore your approach to hitting with questions such as these:

- Can you keep your head in the game even after consecutive strikeouts or making an error in the field? That is, how do you handle holiday mishaps without falling back into old habits for an extended period of time?

- What is your approach to vacations, eating chocolate, or getting back on track after a binge?

- Do you continue to exercise even when you're struggling with your eating?

You may hit homeruns with the amount of weight you lose—or you may hit singles. The important part is staying in the game without giving up, and continuing to focus on your health while balancing other parts of your life.

As previously discussed, bariatric surgery is a bigger bat, so to speak, and only certain folks should use it. Surgery is not better in all cases, and many of you will be using a smaller bat. However, all great baseball players have common characteristics to their swing, no matter what size bat they use. Along those same lines, we need certain attributes for successful weight management.

Check Your Weight, AND Keep Your Eye on Behavior

Research shows that frequent weighing helps prevent relapse. People who keep weight off tend to step on the scale at least weekly. By comparison, those who are unsuccessful with their weight often view the scale as a tripwire that punishes them if they take a step in the wrong direction. They weigh when they know they're following a safe path, but avoid the scale when they veer a little off course.

In previous chapters we covered ways to adjust our thinking in order to view the scale as a dependable friend giving us positive feedback to help correct our course. I encourage each client to use these skills and eventually reach a point of weighing regularly, especially when the body reaches a natural plateau after weight loss.

Even though regular weighing is extremely helpful to prevent relapse, weight doesn't tell the whole story about progress. For example, a 40-pound weight loss can represent different things for different people, based on starting weight and weight-loss treatment. If a 400-pound man has gastric bypass surgery, loses 40 pounds, and then has a six-month weight plateau, he has probably relapsed. His lack of expected weight loss tells us there are problems. He probably returned to unhealthy eating patterns that might include high-fat snacks, sweet tea, or fast food.

Let's compare this surgery patient to a woman who is less overweight, lost 40 pounds, and kept it off for three years without bariatric surgery. In her case, the weight plateau is probably a sign that she's following a healthy eating plan and regular physical activity—even if she's still 30 pounds overweight by medical definition. Her metabolism and appetite have adjusted to her new weight, so the plateau isn't necessarily a sign of unhealthy habits.

As the previous figure suggests, most people who lose weight are still considered overweight or obese by body mass index (BMI), a simple weight to height calculation. It's crucial for you to remember that maintaining weight loss has many health benefits, even if the charts still indicate you're overweight. Just because your weight plateaus at a number higher than you desire (or a BMI chart recommends) doesn't mean you're doing something wrong or you relapsed into old behavior. The only way to truly evaluate *how* you're doing is to look at *what* you're doing.

> *Maintaining weight loss has many health benefits, even if the charts still indicate you're overweight.*

We can rarely define weight-related relapse with one behavior, so you need to look at many daily decisions when examining your lifestyle.

Comparing eating behavior relapse to drug abuse gives us another way to look at this concept. With drug use, an addicted person relapses when he returns to using drugs. It's usually black or white—he's either clean or relapsed. Although the addict often starts behaving in ways that predict relapse, we define relapse with specific behavior: He's using again.

Weight management is different because the behaviors aren't black and white. Eating cheesecake can be part of an overall healthy eating plan—or it may be one of many signals that someone has relapsed into old patterns. For successful long-term weight loss, you need to maintain a variety of healthy practices such as regular exercise, portion control, balance between food groups, and limiting calorie-dense foods.

Frequent weighing is a simple and helpful way to create a centerpiece for your relapse prevention plan. But remember, we weigh ourselves to become more aware of our behavior. And behavior should be the focus of our plan to get back on track when we struggle.

Identify and Plan for High-Risk Situations

If you have an important work-related meeting at eight o'clock in the morning and a snowstorm is supposed to hit your area at 4:00 a.m., what would you do? If you're planning a long car trip, how do you prepare? What if your child complains of a stomachache before bed? Experienced snowy weather residents, veteran travelers, and wise parents understand each of these situations is high-risk for something undesirable to happen. Being on time for a meeting may require getting up early to shovel the driveway and allow for a longer commute. An experienced traveler packs in advance and has the car serviced before a long trip. When a child complains of stomach problems before bedtime, parents soon learn to prepare for a possible upchuck in the middle of the night. (My mother sent us to bed with "puke sacks," and my wife's family used bowls, which makes me leery of eating soup when visiting them).

> *When it comes to exercising and eating the right foods, high risk situations are all around us.*

My point is, most of us know how to identify, plan, and prepare for high-risk situations in our lives. We know what works and what doesn't. Based on experience, we change our approach over time.

When it comes to exercising and eating the right foods, high risk situations are all around us. What events jeopardize your weight management goals? Weekends, vacations, holidays, celebrations, stress, and any life transition can lead to lapses and even full-blown relapses. Think about the last time you lost weight and then began regaining it. What was going on? If similar things happened again, how could you prepare beforehand and how could you handle things differently?

Some high-risk situations are small, day-to-day events that throw us off course. Matt told me he had an issue with overeating cashews at work. He always kept a can of nuts in his desk drawer in case he worked late or missed lunch. But during normal work hours when he did have lunch, the cashews presented a problem. When things got hectic or he felt a bit hungry he'd help himself to "just one handful." That small snack turned into mindlessly picking at cashews all afternoon until the entire can was empty. He could keep other foods at his desk without a problem, just not cashews. He said cashews weren't a problem at home. But the combination of his work environment, plus cashews, created a perfect storm for Matt.

Other people may be overcome by shopping when hungry, having homemade cookies at home during a stressful time, driving with snack food in the passenger seat, and a dozen other scenarios that can be avoided by planning ahead.

Other high-risk situations are unavoidable. Only a hermit could totally avoid social events that challenge healthy eating. Still, we need to anticipate problems whenever possible and have a plan to stay on track. Every stressful event you prepare for is helping you develop skills to handle future situations, even the toughest ones. The longer you practice those coping behaviors and the more natural they feel, the less likely you are to fall apart when your life changes.

Realistic Expectations

Our hospital-sponsored weight loss program includes 20 sessions over seven months. During the first ten sessions patients see a physician and a behavioral specialist every week to work on specific nutrition, exercise, and psychological goals. The appointments spread out to every other week after the first ten weeks. Patients often lose 10 to 15 pounds during the first month and another 5 to 10 pounds during weeks six to ten. If you needed to lose 60 pounds, this would put you one-third of the way to your goal — an exciting accomplishment.

This is when expectations rise. Buoyed by their success, many clients say, "I'll bet I can lose another forty pounds during the second half of the program. I just need to keep working hard, get a little more consistent with my exercise, and I think I can do it."

I never like raining on anyone's parade but our conversation usually ends with at least a few sprinkles. The goal is possible, but highly unlikely for a variety of reasons, including metabolic changes, neurochemicals affecting appetite, and psychological factors such as restraint fatigue. What will happen to these folks if they only lose five more pounds or no weight at all in the next ten sessions? What if they gain back five pounds?

When our expectations are too high and we miss a goal it's easy to lose sight of what we've already accomplished. Losing 20 pounds and gaining back five is still progress and will improve your health. Imagine if every time you lost weight and regained just a little of it, you could view this as a success, not a fatal setback to your plans.

Suppose you get through a season of travel softball for your daughter, an injury to your back, the holiday season, or long work hours with only a few pounds gained? In my book, that's a big accomplishment. Good for you!

Of course you don't want to ever regain *any* weight, but it will happen at some time. People regain a little weight with nonsurgical interventions, the use of appetite suppressants, and after bariatric surgery. Expecting it to never happen is unrealistic and leads to anxiety-provoking fear. If you get married, you'll argue with your spouse. If you have children, they will misbehave. Invest in the stock market and sometimes you'll lose money. Lose weight, and a portion of it will be regained. If we accept this as normal and treatable, you needn't fear it—especially if you have a back-up plan.

Contingency Planning

Fire safety is a big deal where I work. Fires in a hospital can be devastating, so our administrators work hard to prevent them. They also consider worst-case scenarios and give us contingency plans in case of a fire, natural disaster, or other danger. We can do the same thing with weight loss. Just as fire alarms and smoke detectors give warnings of fire, we can set up an early detection system for danger in our weight management efforts.

At the beginning of a relapse your weight begins drifting upward, often without your awareness. Perhaps you're distracted by a change in your life that takes precedence over diet and exercise. Before you know it, your body adds ten pounds. This is when your bathroom scale turns into a smoke alarm: "Danger! Weight gain!"

Frequent weighing can help avoid this scenario. When the patients I work with decide to stop treatment after successful weight loss, we discuss the future: How they'll recognize trouble and what they'll do to self-correct. Weighing ourselves is a simple, easy way to sound an alarm that signals us to take action.

The action part of this process is slightly different for each person. Often the first bullet point after *In case of fire*: is *remain calm*. The same goes for a slip in your weight management. Stay calm, and problem-solve. Fretting over weight gain, putting yourself down, and overreacting will not help. Ignoring the problem won't help either. Stay calm and follow the rest of the plan you created. Preventing a slip from becoming a catastrophic fall usually contains such elements as self-monitoring your diet, planning meals and physical activity, and examining the thinking process that led to this point.

Sometimes you may need professional help to get back on track, such as visiting with a registered dietitian, a physician, a therapist who specializes in weight management, or a personal trainer. The use of appetite suppressants may also be part of the plan.

Neil lost 60 pounds in a year of treatment and decided, because of finances and a one-hour drive to our center, that he would try to maintain this weight loss (and hopefully lose another 20 pounds) without his individual appointments. We created a contingency plan for him based on these warning signs:

- Exercising less than three times per week.
- Drinking alcohol more than twice per week, or to excess.
- Snacking between meals when not hungry.
- Weight gain.
- Current weight: 200; Weight below 205 is acceptable.

Neil's Specific Plan:

- Weigh daily.
- If weight hits 205 for three consecutive days, I will begin recording my food again to determine the problem and/or increase my awareness of eating.
- I will do this until my weight and behavior are stabilized.
- If I'm unable to do this or if my weight hasn't returned to less than 205 within two weeks, I will email you with a more specific plan.

- My note will include a three-day meal plan and my plan for exercise over the next three days. I will do this for two weeks.

- If this isn't successful, I'll make an appointment to come back to the center.

- If at any time my weight hits 210, I'll make an appointment right away.

As I write this, I'm reminded that I haven't heard from Neil. I hope that means he's doing well. I'll give him a call and report back in a later chapter.

Do Something Quickly to Get Back on Track

Larry was a great guy; a caring soul who along with his wife had raised three biological children and had numerous foster kids, four of whom they adopted. He loved conversation and had a great interest in other people. My role was to help *him* get a handle on his diabetes, lose weight, and get physically active. I often redirected our conversation to strategies Larry could use to make his life healthier.

One day after about nine months of treatment Larry said, "You know what I've learned since starting in this program?

"What's that?" I asked.

"First I've learned that I screw up every day. I make a poor food choice or I have two drinks when I only planned to have one. I miss planned workouts. I deviate from my plan. But I already knew that before I came to see you. What I really learned here is how to handle my screw-ups. I used to get so discouraged I'd go way off track and then make a plan to start over at a later time. I don't do that anymore."

"So how do you handle it now?"

"As soon as I realize what I've done, I ask myself, "What can I do, right now, to get back on track? And then I do something right away."

"Can you give me an example?" I asked.

"The other night, I had a second drink when I only planned to have one. So I took the dog for a walk. Last Friday I ate a doughnut at the office. I wasn't happy about it. Well, I was sort of happy while I ate it, but not pleased with my decision. I took three minutes and wrote down what I was going to eat for lunch and dinner. Right away I started feeling better about myself and my ability to stay on track. Psychologically, this is much easier than getting *way* off track and then trying to overcompensate. I feel like I've become pretty good at making corrections when I mess up."

Practice Messing Up

Yes, you read correctly, and not everyone agrees with me on this one. Practice messing up--eat junk food? Isn't that like telling an alcoholic to drink just a little bit?

I wouldn't give this advice to an alcoholic, but food isn't the same as alcohol. We have to eat in order to survive. Alcohol is optional and we can choose to totally *abstain* from it. When it comes to food, we must *manage* our diet in one way or another. Labeling foods unhealthy and then totally abstaining from all of them can be an overwhelming and unnecessary task. Where should you draw the line? The list can become endless and leads to frustration. You start feeling guilt about eating from the wrong list, like an addict who hijacked his recovery.

> *Wouldn't it be nice to enjoy not-so-healthy food without feeling like you messed up each time? The only way to do this is to practice.*

Wouldn't it be nice to enjoy not-so-healthy food without feeling like you messed up each time? Practicing is the only way to do this. I've met many folks who view certain foods as *bad* and when they eat that food they are *being bad*. They associate ice cream, fudge, or gooey chocolate chip cookies with lack of willpower or being out of control. Over time this view becomes part of a self-fulfilling prophesy. When they eat something loaded with fat and sugar they view themselves as out of control. As a result of these beliefs, they eat the dessert in an out-of-control way. Guilt prevents them from enjoying the food and sometimes they shame themselves back to eating only from the healthy-food list. At other times, especially when their defenses are down, they veer way off track. It's sort of a shame.

It's true that we don't need Ho Hos, Doritos, or bacon double-cheeseburgers served between two doughnuts, and it may be a good idea to add a few items to the "Food I Refuse to Put in My Mouth" list. Yet some foods give us a great deal of pleasure, even though they have little redeeming value. We can make these foods fit into an overall healthy diet. Here's what happened during a meeting with a patient named Theresa:

Theresa smiled at me and said, "So let me get this straight. My assignment for this week is to eat chocolate?"

"It is," I said. "Look, you really enjoy chocolate and you don't want to entirely cut it out of your diet, right?"

"That would be accurate."

"So, to me, it makes sense to practice eating it so you have a sense of control and confidence when you do."

Several times per week, usually on the weekends, Theresa ran errands and would have an intense craving for chocolate. Sometimes she resisted the cravings but at other times she gave in—and gave in big time. With urgency in her step and intention in her eyes she'd grab a bag of chocolate miniatures at the self-checkout line. She knew she was *breaking the rules* so she had to do it fast, before logic could prevail. She would then get in her car and rapidly devour half the bag before slowing down. Defeated, she would finish the bag of chocolates while sitting in the parking lot of the grocery store. She discarded all evidence—receipts, wrappers and the candy bag---before driving home, hoping to forget anything out of the ordinary happened. Our conversation went something like this.

"So tell me how much you enjoy these bags of chocolate," I said.

"At first it tastes very good, I guess, but it's also like getting rid of a craving."

"So it's taking something unpleasant away, the craving, as well as giving you pleasure?"

"Exactly. At times the chocolate isn't as good as I think it's going to be. It reminds me of how I used to crave cigarettes, even though I didn't always enjoy smoking. Sometimes I liked it quite a bit, but sometimes I smoked just to get relief from the craving."

"That makes sense," I said. "Now I want you to imagine that eating chocolate is okay, for just a minute. Maybe you can think of chocolate as God's gift just for you! It's not wrong in any way for you to eat it."

"That sounds nice," she said, as she opened her eyes wide and wrapped her thumb and index finger around her chin.

"You don't have to fight *wanting it* with *I shouldn't have it*," I said.

"I like that idea," she said, nodding her head.

"If you felt this way, how much chocolate would you eat before you stopped?"

"Oh, I've never thought of chocolate that way. I don't know exactly, but probably half of the bag or less."

"Why less than you eat now?"

"I eat the second half of the bag because I've already messed up and it's sitting right beside me in the passenger's seat."

"Now I want you to consider the value of the chocolate to you. Let's use an analogy: When is the last time you bought a car?"

"I bought one two years ago," she said.

"Was it new or used?"

"It was new, the only new car I've ever owned."

"How did you make that decision?"

She shrugged. "I thought about what I wanted and how much I was willing to pay for it."

"So cost was a consideration?"

"Absolutely."

"Let's think about your chocolate this way," I said. "You want it, but there are costs, such as calories, how you feel after eating, etcetera. How many calories are you be willing to spend to get what you want?"

"The first seven or eight miniatures are really enough for me. I would feel like I got my chocolate fix and it was in my budget. I think they're about 30 calories each, so I would spend 200 to 250 calories."

"Would you feel deprived?"

"I'm not sure, but I don't think so. I'd actually feel like I got what I wanted in two different ways—I got some chocolate and I stayed within a reasonable calorie budget. Sure there's a little restriction; if I were God I'd make chocolate calorie free!"

"What we just did together—can you do it on your own this week?

"You mean eat seven or eight pieces of chocolate?"

"Well maybe, but I believe the way you think about chocolate is the first step."

"Okay, but do you really want me to eat some after I've thought about it?"

"I think practice may help you, but I'm not sure if buying a whole bag of chocolate is the best way to approach this. Even if we work on your thoughts, having a whole bag beside you is difficult to resist. Do you think you could deal with the whole bag?"

Laughing, "No; I think it would be too hard for me to stop."

"Do you like any candy bars as much as you like the miniatures?" I asked.

"Actually I do. I guess in my mind I'm always telling myself I'll just eat a few pieces per day, so I buy the minis."

"How about if we plan on buying a candy bar this week?"

"You're giving me permission?" she asked.

"Yes, but can you give yourself permission?"

"I think so."

"I also want you to try to eat slowly and enjoy it. Take small bites and savor each one. You might even glance at your watch and see how long it takes you to eat it like this."

"Should I do this each time I have a craving?"

"What do you think is the best approach?"

"I don't think that's a good idea, because what if I have a craving every day or twice per day?"

"Good point. You've used a lot of good methods to ride out cravings in the past. I suggest you continue using strategies like distraction, waiting 30 minutes before you decide whether or not to eat, or distracting yourself with a fun activity." I paused to let my words sink in, then added, But I still think you need to practice eating chocolate in a healthier way. Let's get specific about how you can have a guilt-free rendezvous with your candy bar."

"I think Saturday afternoon is the best time. I would enjoy it most because, although I'm running errands, I'm not in a hurry. "

"Where do you want to eat it?"

"I know people say you should eat at the table, but I just don't think that will work for me. I like taking a break in my car. I tend to associate eating in the car with a binge, so maybe if I practice eating less while in the car it won't be such a problem in the future. Can I try it in my car? I'll just sit in the grocery store parking lot and listen to the radio—I won't drive and eat."

"That sounds reasonable for now," I said. "I do think you may like eating in the car because it's private and somewhat secretive, but we can talk about that later. Let's give it a shot for this week."

Theresa continues to work on controlling her chocolate intake. Many times her goal is to abstain from chocolate altogether. But our practice with moderation has increased her confidence in eating smaller amounts of one of her favorite foods. When she eats chocolate according to her plan, she experiences guiltless pleasure and satisfaction. She also maintains her 30-pound weight loss.

The best practice is one you think through ahead of time. We all have many activities, like vacations, holidays, weekends at the lake, or running errands that make managing weight more difficult. If we want to become better at loosening but not letting go of the reins, we need a plan before we practice. When we make a plan and follow it, we feel like we're on track—which is crucial when the plan involves deviating somewhat from our usual healthy eating and physical activity regimen. I caution you against a common error related to practicing eating the foods we crave: rationalization. It's tempting to start viewing all our dietary indiscretions as practice, when in fact they aren't. Healthy practice requires forethought rather than an explanation after the fact. Your plans should be somewhat systematic with specific and measurable goals. After the practice, evaluate your experience and plan for the next session.

Looking for Lessons

I was wrong, I made a mistake, my plan didn't work and your idea was better. Those are hard phrases for me to say—and words my wife loves to hear.

Life is filled with learning experiences, and the more we try to do, the more we learn. Stretching ourselves brings the risk for failure—but we often learn more from failure than from success. As Henry Ford said, "Failure is the opportunity to begin again more intelligently." When we use failure to make adjustments, we're still making progress. And so it is with weight management. When you give in to food temptation or stop exercising after an exhausting week, it's tempting to forget the whole thing and start over. But if you start over without evaluating what went wrong, you're likely to make the same mistakes again.

After a few weeks off for the Christmas holidays, many of my clients come into the office and say, "I need to get back on track." They lay out plans to get to the gym on a regular basis, eat "clean," and start recording their food again.

I agree with getting back on track, but I also ask them to review what happened so they can be more prepared next season. In fact, I often ask patients to write about their holiday experience: What went well, what didn't work, and how they could handle it better. These holidays come every year, so the temptation is predictable. For many people the "holiday eating season" begins before Halloween with trick-or-treat candy and lasts until January. That's two months, or one-sixth of the entire year. It makes sense to learn from the previous year and develop a plan that will lead to a guilt-free and enjoyable season.

> *"Failure is the opportunity to begin again more intelligently."*
>
> *–Henry Ford*

Chapter 13

Someone is Watching—and You Want Them To

A RECAP OF my workweek reminds me that social support is critical to relapse prevention.

- Last night I joined an exercise class for bariatric surgery patients. As we worked on a cardio routine some people were exactly in step with the leader, while others, like me, struggled to follow her. Nobody cared. Betty, who had her surgery eight years ago, worked out beside Jason who had surgery six weeks ago. A lady six months post-op brought her husband who had surgery a week ago. He sat and watched us, planning to join the class in a few weeks. Matt, a single guy, has been a regular in this group for five years.

- Although he met the weight qualifications, George chose to lose weight without bariatric surgery. This week he showed up for an individual weight management session after being away for a month. His doctors are trying to understand why his painful medical condition doesn't respond to treatment as expected.

"The pain is excruciating, but I'm on the upswing," he told me.

"Many people will let these types of things weaken their determination, but not you. Why did you decide to come in today?" I asked.

"I'm not giving up. I know I've had a lot of health problems, but I won't quit. I need the accountability and support you guys offer. I really appreciate having a place to come that reminds me of why this is important."

- A mother and her 300-pound 14-year-old son, Tristen, started treatment.

"I think we know what to do, but we just can't seem to pull it together and keep it together," his mom told me. "We need support so we can work with each other and stay accountable for our goals."

"What about you, Tristen? Why did you decide to show up tonight?" I asked.

"I want to play basketball this year for my school, but I can't run up and down the court without getting tired. Although I can shoot, I'm too slow. Like Mom said, we need somebody to coach and encourage us, so we don't quit like before."

- I facilitated a bariatric surgery support group.

"Please introduce yourself and tell us why you decided to come tonight," I said as we began our meeting. Person after person revealed they needed support. As I asked them to tell me a bit more, I heard:

"You guys understand."

"I feel comfortable talking about my struggles here."

"I don't feel judged."

"I can't get away with any BS in this group."

One member apologetically wept as she explained she lost her mother three months ago and reverted to emotional eating, gaining 20 pounds. Others chimed in, explaining how they recovered from similar lapses. They encouraged her to not give up. Toward the end of the meeting, several people mentioned the importance of forgiveness in their weight management process.

"We often think about forgiving others or asking God for forgiveness—but we have to forgive ourselves," one man added.

I was amazed that most of the attendees had surgery over five years earlier and several were almost 15 years post-op. They still came to the group because weight management is hard and almost impossible to do alone. Even many years later, they still need support.

- I also spoke to Neil, the guy who lost 60 pounds, going from 260 pounds to around 200 during twelve months of treatment. If you recall, he decided to try and manage things on his own, so we developed a specific contingency plan to help him prevent relapse. Until yesterday I hadn't spoken to him since his last visit six months ago, so I called him.

"Doctor Creel, what's going on?" he answered in his usual upbeat tone.

"I'm just calling to check in on you—I want to see how you're doing with your weight-loss goals."

With his usual laidback attitude, he responded in a surprised but friendly manner, "Oh man, thanks so much for calling, that's awesome. I'm doing good man, how are you?"

Neil sort of has a "cool factor" about him, making communication easy. "Things are good here, too," I said, sounding less hip, I'm sure.

"Oh, wow, well I've been doing pretty well since I stopped coming in. I actually lost another five pounds or so and then Thanksgiving rolled around and you know, I just relaxed a bit, drank a little too much and gained about ten pounds. I actually took about five of those pounds off and then Christmas and family get-togethers and all of that hit. I put on some more weight and actually hit 210. I said, that's my limit and have been doing well since. I'm back down to between 200-205 and I'm feeling good. I just have to keep weighing and make adjustments when my weight heads in the wrong direction. The exercise is still happening. I religiously use my elliptical and I'm thinking about adding strength training."

"It sounds like the scale and your exercise equipment are your friends!"

"Absolutely. I still struggle sometimes with eating cheeseburgers and drinking too much around the holidays or when I hang out with my friends, but you know, I don't feel good when I do that. I just keep reminding myself of that."

"Is there anything we can do to help out?"

"Not right now, but I may come next month just to check in and have some accountability. I really appreciate your call."

"Well, thanks for talking with me, and congratulations on your success. I look forward to seeing you next month, Neil."

Even though Neil didn't follow our contingency plan to perfection, he's doing a lot of things right. He continues to weigh himself and assess the behaviors that lead to weight gain. Our conversation told me he was concerned about weight gain, but didn't get overly upset about it. Instead, he took a practical approach. Sure, he could have had a more specific plan for his deviations around the holidays, and perhaps in time he'll respond a bit quicker to weight gain, but things didn't move too far out of control before he got back on track. His response to my call shows the importance of support for anyone who wants to maintain weight loss. I hope Neil will make it back to the office so we can provide ongoing help.

Humans are social creatures. Solitary confinement is punishment. Children placed in timeout don't like it, because even negative attention is better than being away from the action. Trying to manage your weight without the help of others, can feel like solitary confinement at times—like a continual timeout when everyone else is living a full life while you're stuck in a corner because of some indiscretion or personal weakness. When it comes to something as challenging as managing your weight, feeling alone in a crowd increases your chances of relapsing.

For most of us, the default is to fall prey to unhealthy food and an inactive lifestyle. Having the right kind of support can protect you from pitfalls and inspire you when times get tough.

Perhaps you're already surrounded by people who help with your weight loss efforts. Thank them. Others of you are surrounded by people who want to help but aren't good at it. And some of you don't have anyone to help with your journey.

For those of you who have *Dennis the Menace* supporters (want to help, but seem to make things worse), there is hope. Although it requires a little work, being an effective weight manager requires communication with the people around us. Tell your willing supporters what they can do to help, rather than complaining about how their *help* is annoying. If a person's heart is in the right place he'll listen to you and try to adjust his approach.

Remember that positive reinforcement goes a long way. If your husband every once in a blue moon does something that supports your efforts, tell him exactly what he did and why it helped you. On the other hand, when he tries to assist you with an unhelpful comment such as, "Is that something you should eat?" try hard to communicate you appreciate his willingness to help. Instead of losing your temper, coach him in what to say or do when he notices you eating something that isn't healthy. If you want him to say nothing, let him know that. Over time a caring spouse, friend, or even a professional will get better at providing support when you provide them with feedback and gentle instructions.

If you don't have adequate support or feel as if you need more than your friends and family can reasonably provide, consider joining a group of like-minded people such as:

- Weight Watchers
- TOPS (Take off Pounds Sensibly)
- Overeaters Anonymous
- Hospital sponsored bariatric or general weight management support groups
- A walking club
- Fitness classes
- Cycling clubs
- Recreational sports
- Online support groups

Although the above suggestions can lead to friendships with people who are interested in fitness and healthy weight, you can also find kindred spirits in social activities without a health theme. People can be supportive even if they don't share all your health interests. Volunteering and becoming involved with local groups is a great alternative to pleasure or stress eating and may lead to friendships that will help with your weight management. A quick internet search for volunteer opportunities will show you many ways to get involved, including:

- The United Way
- The Red Cross
- Animal rescue organizations
- Retirement communities
- Hospitals
- Churches
- Battered women's shelters
- Food pantries and soup kitchens
- Coaching youth sports
- Homeless shelters

- YMCAs
- Political campaigns
- Event volunteering
- Schools
- Boys and Girls Clubs

If you're like me, your life already seems full and getting involved with a group may sound overwhelming. Even friendships may be a challenge because of your busy life. If so, this busyness probably makes it harder to manage your weight. Are there responsibilities you can let go of so you have time for true friendship? Is perfectionism keeping you in an overwhelmed state so you don't have time to connect with other people? We all have different needs when it comes to human interaction, but everyone benefits from meaningful relationships—if we slow down and make time for them.

Social anxiety: Getting in your own way.

Maybe you have the time and interest to make new friends, but you feel embarrassed about your body. Social anxiety is common among people who are overweight. I wish it wasn't true, but weight bias is a common social phenomenon. Throughout your life you may have been treated differently and stigmatized because of your size. Some of you have been bullied, ignored, or overtly criticized. As if that isn't enough, you've had to deal with an appearance-obsessed culture that accepts fat jokes even as race, sexual identity, religion, and disabilities are off limits.

First of all, I'm sorry. Secondly, *everyone* doesn't judge or criticize you. The more we fear rejection the more reserved we become, holding back and protecting ourselves. It turns into a vicious cycle: Someone hurt me—I'll keep my distance—I can't make friends because I keep my distance. But as we avoid becoming close to others we miss out on relationships with people who care about us, no matter our size. I often ask clients why they're so worried about what insensitive people think about them. Are these the folks you want to impress? While you're chasing approval from these people, you're missing the ones who are willing to hold your hand through tough times.

Gina, a smart, bubbly, 32-year-old, has never married, although she's an independent professional who would someday like to tie the knot with the right guy. She often pointed out to me that being nearly 100 pounds overweight is a non-starter for the guys she'd like to date. I was a bit skeptical about her beliefs, and it seems I was on to something.

A short time after one of these relationship conversations, Gina spent a weekend out of town helping a few of her girlfriends staff an exhibit at a technology-related conference. On the second day of work her friends began teasing Gina about the guy who was flirting with her.

"What guy?" Gina said.

"You know, the dark haired, tall guy who's always with his two buddies. What's his name... Josh? He's come by like four different times. He's the only person who called any of us by name the entire weekend."

"Oh, please! He's just bored and being friendly," Gina said.

"You wait, he'll stop by again later."

Three hours later one of Gina's friends spotted the same three guys walking toward their booth again. "Heeere comes Josh," she said.

As they approached the ladies, Josh was the first to speak — and he spoke to Gina. "Hey Gina, how late are you going to be here tonight?"

"I don't know, the crowd's starting to thin out. We'll probably be here until six or so, don't you think?" she said as she looked at her friends.

"Do you ladies have any plans for dinner?" Josh asked.

Surprised by his question, Gina looked at her friends who were trying to keep their I-told-you-so smiles from becoming laughter. "Um...I don't think so," Gina looked back toward Josh.

"Would you like to meet us at the Mexican restaurant across the street at about seven o'clock?"

As Gina told me this story, she said the experience made her realize that totally focusing on weight caused her to believe she'd never meet someone interested in her. Although she still believes her weight is a barrier, guys like Josh find her interesting. Gina and Josh didn't maintain a long-distance relationship, but after meeting him she began letting go of the idea that no man will be attracted to her if she weighs more than 150 pounds. Gina also began telling me how her feelings about size made her more reserved in her career and she probably missed opportunities.

"It's possible that people judged me because of my weight, but I don't even know for sure because I didn't try—I was scared to apply for a different job or seek a promotion. My weight caused me to think I wasn't good enough or smart enough." She paused to think for a few moments. "Now I realize how I've been getting in own way," she said, with renewed determination to change her thinking.

Everyone needs something a little different when it comes to finding support for weight management. Even an occasional visit with a professional can boost your confidence and help with your journey. If you decide to do this, choose someone who has knowledge and experience with weight management. Equally important is your personal connection with your new counselor. Can you be completely honest without fear of judgment? Does he or she listen well? Does this person have the ability to understand your situation and partner with you on your next steps? Registered dietitians, therapists, physicians, or fitness professionals are potentially good collaborators.

Chapter 14

Your Recipe for Success

THIS CHAPTER PRESENTS an overview of everything we've discussed about weight management. I hope you'll be reminded of ideas that resonated with you, and perhaps you'll decide to reread a particular chapter.

As I wrap up what I have to say on the subject of weight, I'm reminded of a valuable lesson from my parents: *Just like money and status, weight isn't the most important thing in life. A number on the scale is just that.*

Hopefully you know what's most important in your life. Maybe your list would include family, faith, feeling at peace, close friendships, feeling your life has purpose, or leaving the world a better place. Perhaps you just want to be happy, calm, or live without physical or emotional pain. Maybe you've discovered that unhealthy eating is tightly connected to something on your list and you want to change that. You can.

Weight Loss is a Holistic Process

You may have told yourself, "If I can just lose X number of pounds, I'll be happy." I'm reminding you that weight loss alone will not lead to sustained happiness. It won't give you a ticket to the Magic Kingdom where all your wishes are granted. Instead, our weight often changes as a result of finding inner peace. When our lives are purposeful, we can view health as a vehicle that takes us where we want to go. Without this perspective, the positive feelings we get from weight loss quickly fade or become overshadowed by the chaos of life. When everything competes for our attention, eventually we lose focus on weight. But living purposefully lets us integrate health into the most valuable parts of our lives. The competition between health and other life demands comes to a halt and we're no longer managing weight in a vacuum: We've connected it to things that are already important to us.

The path of weight management has many obstacles. We each have a body we were born with, complete with genetic factors that can impact our journey. These influences are a normal part of the trip and we can't eliminate them, even when they slow our progress.

Plus, side trails can take us in the *wrong direction*. For example, forever searching for the holy grail of food combinations that will melt away pounds gets in the way of developing a sensible eating style. The most important aspects of weight management are not found in the minutia of the effects of a single food, the time of day you exercise, or whether or not you swear off pasta.

Instead, we succeed by using strategies to create a lifestyle that includes balanced eating and regular physical activity. The best plan will promote health and also embrace your schedule, your likes and dislikes, your personality, and your biological tendencies.

On the other hand, sometimes our lifestyle and personal preferences create so many barriers that it is nearly impossible to fit in healthy eating and exercise. If this is true for you, you may benefit from altering major parts of your life. Making job or relationship changes, and letting go of unhealthy hobbies can create a suitable environment for change. Weight management is not a short-term effort; it's a commitment with some sacrifice. But each sacrifice brings a reward as you lose weight, feel better, look better, and enjoy more activities.

Commitment grows stronger when we focus on benefits and rewards instead of grumbling about what we've given up. Motivation naturally has peaks and valleys, but your journey will be easier—and faster—if you celebrate your success and remind yourself of the reason for daily discipline.

Goals

Setting and achieving goals is a fulfilling experience, but we need to select the right goals because these targets can make or break our attitudes. Realistic, short-term goals are crucial in the early stages of changing behavior. Before focusing on a goal you need to know why it's important. Goals should be specific and measurable, helping us focus on behavior related to weight.

Monitoring

Self-monitoring the food we eat, how much physical activity we engage in, and numbers on the scale are essential for most weight-loss maintainers. These tracking strategies can make you more aware of your relationship with food.

The Pleasure of Eating

Eating is one of the pleasures of life and each of us has a personal relationship with food. As we explore these connections to food, we can address the pleasure aspect of eating. People who manage to lose weight and keep it off have discovered how to stop using food as a main source of pleasure. Instead, they use food to fuel other aspects of their lives that are satisfying and rewarding. Redefining pleasure by considering it in a broad, long-term way can also make your weight management journey more fulfilling.

Flavor isn't the only thing that makes eating a pleasure. We can also enjoy the color, texture, and life giving, restorative properties of what we consume. Learn to eat slowly and mindfully (not while doing other things), so you can savor your food in guilt-free portions.

Change your Thinking

Thinking differently can help us prevent negative emotions and handle them better when they do occur. As a result, changing our thinking can help us manage our weight.

Thoughts lead to behavior. Therefore, much of the hard work of managing weight should focus on our oft-neglected beliefs related to food choices, physical activity and general life challenges. That's why much of this book is dedicated to the relationship between feelings, behavior, and thinking differently.

> *The perfect lifestyle plan is the one you can follow, and the only way to follow it is to have a healthy and willing perspective.*

The perfect lifestyle plan is the one you can follow, and the only way to follow it is to have a healthy and willing perspective. When you develop this point of view, your weight management journey will be characterized by wisdom, patience, persistence and resiliency.

Keeping the Weight Off

Obesity is a chronic, often relapsing condition and the hardest part of weight management isn't losing weight: it's keeping the weight off. That's why I recommend you begin creating relapse-prevention strategies early in your weight management journey.

Your master plan for preventing relapse should include changing your environment, planning for high-risk situations, viewing your behavior as a choice, and perhaps practicing the controlled eating of trigger foods. Other relapse strategies include changing faulty thinking, noticing problems right away and taking action, and seeking help from others. These simple tools will keep you on track.

Medication and bariatric surgery increase the chances for a better outcome, but these interventions aren't for everyone. No matter what approach you and your physician decide is best, behavior change is required. Bariatric surgery is not brain surgery and an appetite suppressant doesn't cause vegetables to float onto plates or put tennis shoes on feet. We still have to heed the voice of wisdom when deciding about food and exercise.

Systems of Change

For permanent change, we need to modify multiple systems within our lives:

- the system of family and work;
- the system of thoughts, beliefs, feelings, and emotions;
- the system we use to define pleasure;
- and the system that dictates how we balance short-term satisfaction with the gratification of working toward long-term goals.

Since you're part of each of these systems, you *can* change them. Recently a patient reminded me that the challenges of managing weight needn't be a struggle. She said, "I don't see the changes I make as hardships—I view them as opportunities."

We have a path in front of us filled with opportunities for self-reflection, overcoming obstacles, getting help when we need it, and changing how we think. Sometimes the path can seem narrow; at other times it feels steep and rocky. Sometimes we stumble and fall, but we can always get up, dust ourselves off, and keep going.

The rewards sometimes lie within moment-to-moment accomplishments; at other times the path takes us to wide open, beautiful spaces. When we look back, we're amazed at what we've accomplished. Looking forward, we're filled with hope for future achievements and the joy that accompanies them.

Your Recipe for Weight Management

Most weight management books end with a recipe section for low-calorie food. I'm following this tradition but in a slightly different way—with a recipe for weight management success:

Recipe for Weight Management Success

Ingredients:
One bunch of balanced eating, marinated daily in physical activity

An ounce of knowledge

One package of purpose

A cup of commitment

A dash of pleasure substitute

Directions:
Mix all ingredients in a large bowl of support, slice into realistic goals, and coat the slices with healthy thinking and resiliency. Sprinkle with awareness. Bake with patience.

Serves:
Yourself, everyone you care about and those that depend on you.

In the appendix that follows, patients and colleagues have provided their own recipes for success. Although book appendices are often ignored, please don't skip over this one. The stories and advice are down-to-earth and powerful. I learned a great deal from them, and I believe you will too.

True Stories

Melinda: The Insightful Registered Dietitian

MOST REGISTERED DIETITIANS have provided nutrition counseling to people who want to lose weight. Melinda Jones has made this a full-time career for nearly 20 years. Being a busy mother of four school-aged children often leaves her preoccupied with class projects, appointments, and after-school sporting events. Despite her hectic schedule, Melinda works hard to practice what she preaches by eating sensibly and staying physically active. Her healthy weight is not a genetic thing by any means. All the women in her family are overweight and she knows she would be also if she became a grab and go, fast food drive through, breakfast skipping, late-night snacking, soccer mom.

When I asked Melinda why she made a career out of weight management, she seemed a bit uncomfortable about discussing a rare topic—herself. She told me she had a desire to serve people and liked the fact that she could *see* the life-changing results of weight loss with her clients. She went on to explain that helping people manage their weight involves creating relationships with them, which gives her work a sense of purpose.

When Melinda first started counseling others, she viewed things more simplistically than she does now. Living her own life and working with thousands of patients has helped her better understand the complex nature of health behavior. She told me, "Too often, life gets in the way. People want to change, but they're barely getting by, just reacting to things that happen." In this context, Melinda has witnessed the destructive power of food.

However, when people commit to changing their lives and becoming intentional about living, instead of just responding to things that happen, food becomes an amazing healer. Melinda's recipe for success isn't what I expected from a typical nutrition professional, but she is exceptional. Although she could outline a healthy meal plan in her sleep, her advice doesn't mention a thing about meals, artificial sweeteners, or probiotics. Instead of giving specific guidelines about food she focuses on the most important characteristics of success:

- People must know why they want to change and it can't be to please someone else.

- Focus on positives things, not on the negative part of lifestyle changes. Sure, we make sacrifices, but we also reap many benefits that we can choose to notice.

- People who are successful do not feel defeated by missing a goal. They set another goal, along with a realistic plan to achieve it.

- Consistency. People who manage their weight repeat many of the same things every day: keep a regular sleep schedule, eat breakfast, set a specific time for exercise, cook at home, and weigh themselves. They aren't overly rigid, but they also don't regularly take "cheat days" or vacations from healthy eating.

- Success is different for each person but it will never be about following an unrealistic diet. Success only happens when people commit to changing the way they live.

Bill: The Experienced Psychologist

Over the years, Bill Hilgendorf has treated many patients with a variety of psychological disorders. He works full-time for a bariatric center and has a small private practice on the side.

Bill is a great listener, with no urgency to jump in and give his opinion. He slides into conversation with caring words or his sense of humor, which often involves a witty play on words. He is a skilled clinician and caring person. I would send a patient or a family member to him without hesitation.

When summing up his recipe for success, Bill referred to the characteristics of the 30 or so patients who serve as mentors to others involved in his program. He noticed these superstars seem to have five things in common. He uses a hand illustration to describe the components of long-term weight management success: The thumb represents what we eat and the four fingers are connected to these choices:

- *Thumbs up* reminds us to choose food that will nourish our bodies and provide energy.

- Tapping your *index finger* gently on your temple can remind you to eat mindfully. Think when you eat. Pay attention to feelings of hunger and fullness rather than simply eating by the clock, eating because food is available, or eating because others are doing it.

- Of course the *middle finger* is physical activity. Sticking your middle finger in the air by itself can lead you to think exercise is a dirty word. But when we look at the middle finger as part of a hand, it's at the center of everything. Without that finger a hand doesn't work efficiently. Without regular physical activity, we're unlikely to lose weight and keep it off. Our focus can be on both regular exercise (working out) as well as staying active during a typical day.

- The *ring finger* is support. Bill describes getting support with the three *I's*.

  Inspirational support: Find people, groups, or activities that motivate you to keep on keeping on. These are often our friends who listen to us, encourage us, or simply provide a shoulder to cry on.

Informational support: Seek out friends, mentors, or professionals who can offer advice or provide education to enhance the weight management journey.

Instrumental support: This type of support comes from people who aren't afraid to get their hands dirty. They help you prepare healthy meals, exercise with you, or babysit your toddler so you can go to the gym regularly.

- The *pinkie* reminds us of small things that make a big difference. They fall under the category of self-awareness and include food and activity tracking, self-weighing, measuring portion sizes, journaling your thoughts, and getting regular feedback from a professional.

Donny and Paula: The Successful Couple

"They don't seem like they've been married 42 years," I said to myself as Donny and Paula told me about their weight management journey. They communicated so well; when they recalled things differently they didn't argue; one of them would just say, "You might be right about that." As they mentioned the rough times, such as Donny's past battles with alcohol, it seemed Paula had truly forgiven him and Donny appeared to forgive himself. I found their relationship refreshing—the way a marriage should be, like good friends.

After they began dating Donny and Paula found out they worked at the same place at the same time and lived in the same apartment as children—at different times, of course. Maybe something supernatural connected them after Paula inherited Donny's old room!

The first time Donny brought Paula home to meet his parents, his mother pulled him aside and told him Paula was overweight—very overweight, as if she thought Donny couldn't see for himself. Paula and Donny both came from alcoholic homes. Donny and his brother ran around the neighborhood unsupervised and had a free-for-all with food.

Paula, on the other hand, compensated by trying to mediate conflict and act appropriately so Dad wouldn't become upset and get plastered. She remembers using food as comfort when she was four years old. As an only child, she had no siblings to insulate her from their dysfunctional home. Being left alone for hours after school gave her unsupervised access to unhealthy food, just like Donny.

As a young couple they fueled each other's dysfunctional relationship with food. They described going to the store to buy pie. They would buy two pies and each of them ate their own in the grocery store parking lot. Donny and Paula realized food was an issue for them, so they began attending Weight Watchers meetings together. Although a step in the right direction, they routinely attended meetings and then headed across the street to an all-you-can-eat buffet where they'd gorge on crab legs with melted butter. "As soon as the meeting was over, our tires were smokin' to get over to the restaurant as fast as we could," Donny told me.

Although they had on and off success with Weight Watchers, they weren't ready to change permanently, yet. However, they were committed to the weekly meeting routine and observing the success and failure of others planted seeds for their eventual metamorphosis. They continued dipping their toes in the water until ten years before our meeting when Paula had bariatric surgery. Donny followed two years later, and their lives have never been the same.

Paula has maintained a 190-pound weight loss, Donny 154. They continue attending Weight Watchers and several bariatric support groups. Each of them shared events that positively and negatively reinforce their healthy behavior. Paula remembers her childhood nickname, Crisco, and wants to stay away from anything that reminds her of that outgrown identity. Danny is still bothered by the fact that a coworker called him Bluto (a.k.a. Brutus from the Popeye cartoon). Both noticed that people began viewing them as smarter when they lost weight. Although they dislike these assumptions, they feel life is much easier at a healthy weight.

Donny says he remembers a man who attended Weight Watchers meetings many years ago before his own bariatric surgery. "I remember telling Paula he had no neck!" But then they noticed the thick-necked man began to lose weight—a lot of weight. They were intrigued by his success and found out he had bariatric surgery. The fact that he could change inspired both of them to consider doing the same. But a year or so after his surgery the man began missing a lot of meetings. They noticed he was regaining weight, and then he stopped coming. One day they saw him around town and it was obvious he'd regained a lot more weight. Donny saw the power of bariatric surgery but he also observed that surgery guaranteed nothing long-term. No-neck man reminded him that surgery won't do all the work. It's only a tool and it's up to him to use it.

Paula and Donny's success is based on more than the fear of regaining weight. They both love the fact that they can move better and they enjoy challenging their bodies with physical activity. Donny is an avid cyclist, training for and completing a one-day 160-mile ride every year. One year he got off course and actually pedaled 184 miles. Paula likes to walk; she challenges herself at the gym and enjoys setting new fitness goals.

Paula told me, before bariatric surgery she thought about food all the time. "That hasn't changed much," she added. But food is no longer what she obsesses about to give her pleasure. Instead, she plans meals to help her live the way she wants. This is a message she tries to relay to others who want to manage their weight.

Giving back to others by helping with their weight management journeys is another motivating factor for this dynamic couple. Attending multiple support groups each month reminds Donny and Paula of their past lifestyle and helps them continue on the right path. Hearing the advice they give others solidifies their commitment to stay on track. Although they agree there's no magic formula for weight loss and everyone's success story is slightly different, I can sum up what they told me in the following way:

- You must be honest with yourself about how you're doing and where you're heading. Data such as the frequency of exercise and numbers on the scale don't lie, so pay attention to that information by weighing daily and planning exercise.

- Don't throw yourself down the stairs because you slip on one step. Nobody's perfect, especially with eating. When you mess up, learn from it and keep pursuing your goals.

- Know your limits. If there is a food that you cannot eat in moderation, no matter how hard you try, keep it out of the house and be willing to give it up. If it's destroying your life, view it as a recovering alcoholic sees alcohol. Paula stated that although it may be possible to learn to eat that food in moderation, ask yourself, "Why is it so important to spend that much energy on one food when you may not succeed? Plus, the attempt at moderation may throw you off track." She advises, "Don't play with fire, and unless you're a firefighter or a hibachi grill master, stay away from it altogether."

- Learn from others. Watch closely as those around you succeed and stumble, and apply those lessons to your journey. This is different than looking at others' experiences to confirm your own ideas. We can always find someone who seems to break the rules and gets by okay, but what do you see with the majority of people who are successful and/or struggle?

- Let go and let God. Some things we can never fix or totally understand. This is especially true when it comes to childhood experiences that leave us scarred, vulnerable, or feeling unlovable. Food is often a convenient, temporary escape from these feelings. Letting go means realizing we are loved and God has a plan for our lives. We all have unique talents and value, no matter our size, our past, or how we *feel*.

- Get support and be support. Find a community that will hold you accountable, help you up when you fall, and laugh with you along the way. As you mature in the process, find a way to give back. Not only will this help others, it will help you stay on track as well.

- Realize the food plan is only a small part of success. Move beyond long lists of food rules and explore your relationship with food.

- Fearing weight regain is normal and okay to a degree, but don't be consumed by fear. Keep it at bay by setting goals that are rewarding when you achieve them. Physical activity pursuits are a good place to start.

Jessica: The Formerly Overweight Physician

Do you ever wonder if your physician has a clue? Time after time he says you need to lose weight, but does he know how hard that is? Has he ever walked in your shoes? Although no two people ever have exactly the same experience, it's reassuring to know that people who give advice truly understand your situation and emotionally connect with what you're trying to achieve. When it comes to managing weight, Dr. Jessica can relate.

As the youngest of three girls and the child of a mother who had a love/hate relationship with food and exercise, Jessica became well-versed in dieting lingo at a young age. Jealousy between her normal weight and overweight sisters taught her that a thin body was something to be coveted. All the while, her mom's on-again-off-again diets led to inconsistency in what food was available at home. At family gatherings the women always talked about food and diets they were on, or about to start. Jessica recalls climbing on top of the bathroom sink so she could have a full-length mirror to determine if her chubby legs looked unattractive in her soccer uniform. She was only 5-years-old.

Her weight history is like a neon sign flashing in her memory bank. When all the fifth graders at her school were weighed as part of fitness testing, Jessica was one of only three girls who topped the 100-pound mark. At that time, in her town, childhood obesity was not as prevalent as it is today, and her size was something she couldn't hide. As a middle schooler she tried to restrict calories and follow the lead of everything she learned about dieting from her family. This led to some yo-yoing of her weight, but soccer was what really prevented her weight from ballooning out of control. Though a bit heavier than the other girls, she was a good player. Lots of practice, games, and all-day weekend tournaments kept her on the move and made it difficult to consume more calories than she burned. She loved the sport and continued playing through high school and even competed at the small university she attended.

But when college soccer ended and Jessica began medical school, things began to change. Long hours of studying, stress, and less physical activity led to steady weight gain. Her family medicine residency only made things worse, demanding even longer hours and more pressure to perform well. By her third year of residency she was 40 to 50 pounds overweight.

Despite gaining weight, Jessica never lost her dieting mentality. If she ate the wrong things, she was aware and felt guilty. She tried to manage her weight, but seemed to be just spinning her wheels. As a physician she knew the dangers of obesity and feared the plight of many women in her family.

During her third year of residency, Jessica's approach to dieting turned on its head. She heard Dr. Michelle May, the author of *Eat What You Love, Love What You Eat* present a different perspective on weight management. Dr. May's non-restrictive, mindful approach to eating taught Jessica to pay attention and eat when she was hungry, slow down, and pay attention to fullness. She became more aware of her relationship with food and learned to avoid emotional eating. She stopped having negative feelings if she decided to eat less-healthy food in moderation. She began exercising because it made her feel good, rather than exercising just to burn off something she shouldn't have eaten.

As a result, Jessica lost 45 pounds over 18 months. Ten years and three kids later, Jessica has maintained her weight without returning to yo-yo dieting or guilt-driven behavior. As a family physician she works closely with her patients, helping them lose weight and maintain their success. Her personal experiences shaped the recipe for success she promotes.

- Stop using food as a consolation for a bad day or as a reward for hard work. Instead, find other rewarding, pleasurable things to do. Jessica encourages people to make a list of ten non-food treats to replace food. Five of them should be quick and easy things that can be "go tos" after a tough day, or a reward for a job well done.

- Cope with problems rather than using food to tamp down negative emotions. Understand what drives your eating and tackle those things head on. Jessica quotes Dr. May and says, "If a trigger doesn't come from hunger, eating will never satisfy it."

- Exercise because it makes you feel good, not to burn off calories.

- Enjoy things in moderation without guilt. Anything forbidden is alluring. Take the power away—everything is permissible, but not beneficial.

- Keep the environment clear of triggers. Even though Jessica doesn't make anything off limits, she suggests keeping high-risk foods out of arm's reach.

- Realize that your approach may need to change in each season of life. Sometimes it's most helpful to focus on planning our behavior, while at other times we have to think more about handling our emotions, being mindful of our reactions, or making the best of a less-than-ideal situation.

Bill: The Practical Personal Trainer

If I wanted to hire a personal trainer, I would choose Bill Dean. He has never been a bodybuilder, followed a diet centered around protein shakes, canned tuna, or egg whites, nor does he have much interest in six-pack abs. He's a fit guy in his mid 40's who believes in an honest day's work, a good laugh, and making a difference in people's lives. His clients range from professional athletes to stay-at-home moms. He's worked with multi-millionaire executives and average wage earners who are making financial sacrifices to get help with improving their health and well-being. Some of Bill's clients come to him tremendously overweight and out of shape, while others are relatively fit and want to stay that way.

Despite missing opportunities to make a quick buck, Bill hasn't conformed to an industry driven by promises to get ripped, turn eyes in a bikini, or serve only those who want to have a "status" trainer.

So what drives Bill? People. He has a knack for tapping into the core reasons people want to get fit or improve their health. When he asks clients about their *why* he tells them to think three levels deep. People want to get healthy, but not just to be healthy; they want to do things, create something, or feel a certain way.

Bill told me people miss out when they compare themselves to others or focus on numbers. He doesn't get fired up about body fat percentages, progress on the scale, or how you compare to others on a fitness test. Numbers are just numbers and they don't mean anything. *Feeling better* means something and so does having more self-confidence or less back pain. It means something when you can sleep better at night or feel less overwhelmed by your busy lifestyle.

Bill illustrated this point with a story about one of his clients who, on days when she isn't training with him, does an indoor cycling class at a local gym. The cycles are connected to an electronic board in the front of the room that displays how much work each cyclist is performing compared to other people in class. This client is a hard worker and leaves the class exhausted; nevertheless, she's usually last on the leaderboard. Focusing on the fact that she's a last place finisher discourages her. She leaves the gym feeling like a boxer knocked out in the final round of a hard-fought contest.

"It makes no sense for her to feel this way," Bill told me. She's up early on a Saturday morning working hard while most people are still in bed. Most of those who *are* up at that hour don't have plans to exercise, or if they do, they won't push themselves like she does. He helps her remain focused on her *why*, which has little to do with seeing her name at the top of a list in a cycling class. Most likely, if she can keep this focus, her fitness will continue to improve and she won't stay at the bottom of the list. But in the grand scheme of things, does it really matter? We can always find stronger, faster, thinner, smarter and richer people than us. On the other hand, there will always be people with fewer of these qualities. We get to choose our comparisons, or decide not to compare at all.

Lastly, Bill commented on how challenging yourself with fitness goals builds resiliency, self-confidence, and mental toughness. Exercising on the days you don't feel like it builds confidence as you realize things that may seem too difficult are actually rewarding. "I've never had a client finish a workout and say, 'I wish I hadn't done it,'" he said. Instead, people are proud of themselves and begin to feel comfortable with excellency.

Bill sees parallels between success in many areas of life and staying fit. Want to have a successful business? Getting and staying fit will teach you persistence. Want to be a better parent? Commit to regular physical activity—it will make you a more patient caregiver. Want to become more confident and self-assured? Challenge yourself in the gym, on the bike, or walking through your neighborhood. In short, Bill's recipe for success with physical activity is as follows:

- Know your *why* (at least three levels deep) and don't get sucked into numbers or comparisons.

- After each workout, remind yourself what you just did, even though you didn't have to do it.

- Dedicate yourself to consistent regular physical activity just as you'd take a medication that keeps you alive.

- When your confidence wanes, let exercise be a reminder that you're capable, functional, and willing to persevere despite life's challenges.

- Don't take yourself or exercise too seriously. Whenever possible, tap into your childlike instincts and make physical activity a playful and enjoyable experience.

- Don't be afraid to hire a trainer, but *own* your fitness. You are the decider, the driver, and the one who explains why your health is worth the effort.

Carol: Actions Not Words

When we met, Carol seemed to be a no-nonsense, just-the-facts kind of woman. During our first few sessions she appeared to endure our back and forth chit-chat about her weight as a requirement to get to the bottom line--a plan. Unlike clients who leave a session saying, "That gives me something to think about," Carol likes to leave saying, "That's something I can use."

During the first four months of treatment we stuck with a well-planned progression to reach her desired weight. We sometimes joked that we were following the manual's instructions, keeping up with the manufacturer's recommended scheduled maintenance, building what she wanted brick by brick.

Over the two years we worked together, Carol broadened her perspective. Although remaining true to her cut-the-fluff approach, she gained an appreciation for stepping back from her detailed goals enough to see the bigger picture of her journey. She became more comfortable sharing what lies behind her eating behavior—her beliefs, emotions, and personality—and learned to appreciate all those behind-the-scenes factors involved with weight management. Combining our discussions and her plans helped Carol identify exactly where she had problems with eating, and she learned what works and what doesn't.

Although we looked for explanations for her behavior, we didn't get bogged down by the *why*. Instead, we chose to look at *how* things happened and then made plans for how she *wanted* things to happen. I learned that Carol is polite, smart, and driven to succeed—someone you'd want on your team. Carol shows great commitment to managing her weight and has an uncanny ability to consolidate information, put a plan together, and then take action.

Carol has never been morbidly obese, but was at an unhealthy weight before starting our sessions. She didn't like the way she felt or the size of her clothes, and she knew unhealthy behavior was to blame. After several years of persistence and remarkable success, she was kind enough to share her recipe for success:

- Track food daily. Carol suggests using a mobile app because most people always have their phones nearby.
- Develop some sort of external accountability. Without someone to check in with, it's too easy to fall back into old behavior, regain weight, and ignore things that contribute to a relapse.

- Weigh daily; it will keep you honest. Stepping on the scale each morning makes it easier to observe day-to-day fluctuations without freaking out about one measurement. You'll learn to look for trends and modify your behavior accordingly.

- Make exercise a priority. If you're always trying to fit exercise between other activities it often gets squeezed out. Instead, plan your days with exercise at the top of the to-do list. Carol suggests taking a fitness class, which also provides social support, or having a set time for your routine.

- Plan and pre-prep meals as much as possible. Use weekends to slice and dice, pre-portion, or cook foods that take a long time to prepare. When your busy week is in full swing, healthy foods are at your fingertips and meals only take minutes to assemble.

- If you drink alcohol, develop strategies to control it. Otherwise your calories can get out of control in a hurry. Not only do the drinks contain calories, but your inhibitions to eating not-so-healthy foods often fly out the window as well. Carol recommends thinking ahead about which social events will lend themselves to drinking and prioritize within a budget of two to three drinks per week.

- Work functions, family pitch-ins, or holiday gatherings can often be part of a downhill spiral for someone trying to manage weight. Bring a healthy dish with you and never take home tempting, high-calorie leftovers.

- Limit desserts. Carol admits to struggling with the sweet stuff. She found that only buying what she wants to eat at one sitting is a good strategy. She rarely bakes because the temptation is too much work to manage.

Joanna: The Wise Weight Manager

Twenty-two years have passed since Joanna hired me as a personal trainer. Unlike some clients, I had no problem getting her to talk about her struggles with weight. In fact, many of her stories straddled the line of *too much information* and left me either bent over with laughter or on the verge of tears. She never shied away from attention and praise, and she also wasn't afraid to earn it. She was a hard worker who wanted me to push her physical limits during training sessions. After an intense workout Joanna would often smile and say, "Look at this!" as she flexed her biceps that were becoming shapely. She was results oriented; her head always seemed full of big ideas and she usually had the intellect, drive, and persistence to accomplish what she set out to do.

Her career was marked by one success after another. She was a visionary who subscribed to the idea that "If it ain't broke, break it, and make it better." She grew an organization beyond anyone's wildest dreams and had a positive impact on hundreds of thousands of people because of it. This drive carried over into her personal life. But the attitude that yielded so much career success led to frustration with her never-ending desire to maintain a healthy weight. She approached each diet full steam ahead with outcomes in mind, often ignoring the fact that this would be a lifelong journey rather than a project she could accomplish and then move on.

Many years ago, near the end of our work together, Joanna wrote about her battle with weight. At the time of her writing she had experienced prolonged success with her weight and had a clear perspective of why weight loss maintenance is so difficult. Through all my moves since then, I kept her notes in a white three-ring binder, tucked in a box of memorabilia. The slight yellowing of the pages and the floppy discs in the notebook remind me of how many years have passed since Joanna asked me to help her become healthier. Despite the passage of time, her words are poignant and represent many beliefs of my current patients.

Do you ever wonder how many tomorrows there are in a lifetime? However many I'm allowed, I was certain I'd used my allotment. If children yell "do-over" quickly enough after making a mistake in jacks, tetherball, hopscotch, or some other game, they get to take their turn again—without penalty. Well, my adult life was constantly a "do-over," but with costly penalties. Every morning I told myself, "Today is the day I'm going to succeed." Success meant I was going to do without. But without *usually turned into* with, *and countless days ended with feelings of failure and a promise that things would be different tomorrow. After 47 years I had accumulated a lifetime of failed yesterdays.*

When I decided to try losing weight just one more time, I convinced myself it was my last chance. My last tomorrow had arrived. I was truly in my all-or-nothing mode of behavior, which is how I lived my life. If I were describing a movie I'd just seen, it was either phenomenal or the worst ever. When I finished a book, it was the most incredible book I ever read or a total waste of time. If I went out with friends, it was the most spectacular evening or truly the pits. My love for my dear husband even fluctuated from unconditional adoration to hate. I was like the children's nursery rhyme, "When she was good she was very good, and when she was bad she was horrid," with nothing in between. I had no middle ground, and this all-or-nothing attitude had proven to be destructive.

How this all-or-nothing attitude relates to weight loss and exercise is easily illustrated. Whenever I began a new diet plan, I stuck to the plan to the letter. I recorded everything I ate. I weighed and measured everything. No one or nothing could make me eat what I wasn't supposed to. I was in my "all" stage. But when I fell off, for God knows what reason, I fell off completely and my "nothing" approach to life kicked in. If I swallowed one morsel of food I wasn't supposed to eat, then I felt I'd failed, and since the day was already screwed up, I might as well eat anything and everything I wanted. My day was ruined, my diet was over, my program was a bust, I was a failure again. Then it would take me weeks, months, sometimes years to get back on a program.

My psychological makeup focused largely on unrealistic expectations. I could convince myself that if I just worked harder at not eating, if I could be more disciplined, I'd look like the fashion models whose pictures plastered my refrigerator door. In addition, I had no realistic timeline. It wasn't unusual for me to expect to lose five pounds a week, or 20 pounds a month. Or 80 pounds in four months. Anything short of that sent me into depression and sometimes derailed whatever more realistic success I was having at the time.

Over the years, Joanna and I occasionally stayed in contact, with several years often passing between communication. Our conversations or brief e-mails were usually more about our families or life changes, not weight. Despite not working together professionally for over two decades, many fond memories of our time together are etched clearly in my mind, as if they happened yesterday. Looking back, I probably learned as much from Joanna as she did from me.

Her willingness to be honest and vulnerable about how weight touched all aspects of her life taught me valuable lessons not found in textbooks or the results section of journal articles. Our training sessions and nutrition counseling rarely felt like work and the questions she asked that I couldn't answer inspired me to learn as much as possible about the field I now enjoy so much. Without our work together, I might not have chosen this career path—and had I chosen it without knowing Joanna, my perspective would be less complete.

Even though I felt a little guilty about not keeping in touch with her, I recently contacted Joanna and asked her if she'd provide an update on her perspective for effectively managing weight. With the same support I remember from years past, she responded, "I'd walk on hot coals for you, Dave."

I've always seen Joanna as a wise woman with strong leadership qualities so I was curious to know if her view on things had changed over the years. She recently retired and is enjoying it much more than she and all her friends and family expected. She cherishes time spent with grandkids who live out of state. She helps her husband with his business and has more time to reflect on her health goals. She told me she doesn't feel 66-years-old and has an image of herself that's only challenged when she sees her reflection. Although she occasionally finds herself staring into the mirror trying to figure out the timeline and progression of an emerging wrinkle or two, her appearance is no longer a driving force to manage her weight.

She described how many people her age were having serious medical problems related to unhealthy lifestyles. Some die prematurely and others simply keep living, but not really. They can't do what they want to do, their schedules are filled with one doctor's appointment after another. Health problems are all they ever talk about. She has no interest in living that way and it is her primary motivation to stay healthy.

So what has Joanna learned after many years of trying to manage her weight, and what advice would she give others? She learned to never say *never* about regaining weight. At the time she wrote the passage above, she was telling herself she'd figured things out and would never be heavy again. But it wasn't that easy. Weight regain is part of the process and if you tell yourself it will never happen, you won't be adequately prepared to handle the situation when it does. If you don't know how to fix a small leak, eventually it becomes much worse and the damage is substantial. Joanna is more pragmatic now than ever before. "My weight will always be a struggle," she told me. Although she wants healthy eating and regular exercise to be as habitual as brushing her teeth, it isn't easy and requires intentional persistence. If Joanna was coaching you about managing weight, you'd become familiar with the following themes:

- Managing weight is not about intelligence. If you're overweight it doesn't mean you're stupid, incompetent, or less of a person. Obesity is a complex condition influenced by genetics, our environment, upbringing, and psychological reactions to life.

- Expect to regain weight after losing it, but have a plan to stop it before the gain is substantial. This plan has to include specific behaviors related to getting back into an exercise routine and eating better. More importantly, your psychological response will determine whether or not you incorporate these behaviors.

- Balance immediate gratification with long-term goals. It's okay to love food but not at the expense of everything else that's important to you—your health, your ability to engage in physical activities you enjoy, or simply feeling energetic.

- Master the art of portion control. Eat slowly, and when you aren't quite full, wait a while and you probably will be. Use a smaller plate and don't eat everything served to you in a restaurant.

- Choose your professional help wisely. Joanna suggests finding someone who understands the basics of nutrition and exercise, but she feels it's even more important to work with someone who has an in-depth knowledge of the psychology of weight management. Work with someone who understands the power of thoughts and can guide you through times of high and low motivation. She encourages you to find someone you can connect with, knowing that person truly cares. If someone tries to fake authenticity, move on to another helper.

- Patience and forgiveness. Weight is something you manage long-term. It's a marathon, not a sprint. Understand that your day-to-day victories with food and physical activity won't immediately show up on the scale. When you mess up, and you will, learn to forgive yourself and have a plan to handle things differently next time.

End Note

I HOPE YOU enjoyed the Recipes for Success in the Appendix, provided by people who shared their weight management experiences—both professional and personal. None of the recipe providers claim to know it all. Like me, my colleagues are still learning new ways to help people improve their health and quality of life. The clients I consulted with admit their imperfections and some still struggle with their weight at times. Although I don't reveal my clients' true identities, I'm grateful for their willingness to help me and you.

To the many clients who were brave enough to share with me their quest for healthier and more meaningful lives—I thank you. Even if I didn't tell your story in this book, you taught me many things. It's humbling to know you trusted me enough to share tears as you worked through tough times. And I loved seeing the ear-to-ear smiles that came with success.

For readers I've never met, I'd love to hear about your weight management experiences. Feel free to contact me through my website, www.drdavidcreel.com, or at: **dbcreel@gmail.com**. You can help me by typing *A Size That Fits* in the subject line of the email. Because computer viruses can cause headaches, I won't open attachments.

(Type *A Size That Fits* in the subject line of your email).

Notes and References

Introduction

- Kraschnewski et al., "Long-term weight loss maintenance in the United States," International Journal of Obesity, 34 (2010): 1644-1654.

- Wikihow.com/Load-Dice illustrates several ways to get an unfair advantage with dice.

Chapter 1

- According to the National Association of Theatre Owners website, the average cost of a movie ticket in 1994 was $4.08.

- While the author completed his Ph.D. and worked for the Pennington Biomedical Research Center, George Bray, MD, Eric Ravussin, PhD, Donna Ryan, MD, Claude Bouchard, PhD, Donald Williamson, PhD, Frank Greenway, MD, Corby Martin, PhD, Robert Newton, PhD, Paula Geiselman, PhD, Catherine Champagne, PhD, RD and many other renowned researchers were employed there. He thanks each of them for providing a fertile environment that helped him grow as a professional.

- While at MUSC, the author worked with Dr. Pat O'Neil, one of the funniest guys he knows. Pat, thanks for writing an entertaining foreword for this book.

Chapter 2

- Online resources such as choosemyplate.gov, eatright.org, and acsm.org provide research-based recommendations for those seeking to improve their diet and fitness.

- Randolph et al., "Potatoes, glycemic index, and weight loss in free living individuals: Practical Implications," *Journal of the American College of Nutrition,* 33 (2014): 375-384.

- Miller et al., "Low-calorie sweeteners and body weight and composition: a meta-analysis of randomized controlled trials and prospective cohort studies," *The American Journal of Clinical Nutrition*, 100 (2014): 765-777.

- Tate et al., "Replacing caloric beverages with water or diet beverages for weight loss in adults: Results of the CHOICE randomized clinical trial. *The American Journal of Clinical Nutrition*, 95 (2012) 555-563.

- Dansinger et al., "Comparison of the *Atkins, Ornish, Weight Watchers,* and *Zone* diets for weight loss and heart disease risk reduction: A randomized trial," *Journal of the American Medical Association*, 293 (2005): 43-53.

- Gaesser et al., "Gluten-free diet: Imprudent dietary advice for the general population?" *Journal of the Academy of Nutrition and Dietetics*, 112 (2012): 1330-1333.

- Fine and Feinman, "Thermodynamics of weight loss diets," *Nutrition and Metabolism*, 1 (2004): 1-8.

- Llewellyn and Fildes, "Behavioral susceptibility theory: Professor Jane Wardle and the role of appetite in genetic risk of obesity," Current Obesity Reports, 2017, 6:38 doi:10.1007/s13679- 017-0247-x.

- Komaroff, "The Microbiome and risk for obesity and diabetes,"*Journal of the American Medical Association*, 317 (2017): 355.

- Sacks, et al., "Comparison of weight-loss diets with different compositions of fat, protein, and carbohydrates," *New England Journal of Medicine*, 360 (2009): 859-873.

- Thomas, et al., "Time to correctly predict the amount of weight loss with dieting," Journal of the Academy of Nutrition and Dietetics, 114 (2014); 857-861.

- Calorie needs vary, based on a variety of factors. The *2015-2020 Dietary Guidelines for Americans* provides a table that estimates calorie needs based on age and physical activity patterns.

- Clinical Practice Guidelines for the Perioperative Nutritional, Metabolic, and Nonsurgical Support of the Bariatric Surgery Patient—2013 Update: Cosponsored by American Association of Clinical Endocrinologists, The Obesity Society, and American Society for Metabolic & Bariatric Surgery.

- Bray et al., "Effect of dietary protein content on weight gain, energy expenditure, and body composition during overeating," *Journal of the American Medical Association*, 307 (2012): 47-55.

- Lichtman, et al., "Discrepancy between self-reported and actual caloric intake and exercise in obese subjects," *New England Journal of Medicine*, 327 (1992): 1893-1898.

- Qibin, et al., "Sugar-sweetened beverages and genetic risk of obesity," *New England Journal of Medicine*," 367 (2012): 1387-1396.

- Rogers, et al., "Does low-energy sweetener consumption affect energy intake and body weight? A systematic review, including meta-analyses, of the evidence from human and animal studies," *International Journal of Obesity*, 40 (2016): 381-394.

- Drewnowski and Bellisle, "Liquid calories, sugar, and body weight," *American Journal of Clinical Nutrition*, 85 (2007): 651-661.

- Willis, et al., "Appetite and gastric emptying differ when fiber is consumed in macronutrient-matched liquid and solid meals," *The FASEB Journal*, 25 (2011): Supplement 328.6.

- Paddon-Jones, et al., "Protein, weight management, and satiety," *The American Journal of Clinical Nutrition*, 87 (2008): 1558S-1561S.

- Swift, et al., "The role of exercise and physical activity in weight loss and maintenance," *Progress in Cardiovascular Diseases*, 56 (2014): 441–447.

- Catenacci, et al., "Physical activity patterns in the National Weight Control Registry," *Obesity*, 16 (2008): 153-161.

- Jakicic,et al., "Effect of exercise on 24-month weight loss maintenance in overweight women," *Archives of Internal Medicine*, 168 (2008): 1550-1559.

- Donnely, et al., "The American College of Sports Medicine position stand. Appropriate physical activity intervention strategies for weight loss and prevention of weight regain for adults," *Medicine and Science in Sports and Exercise*, 41 (2009): 459-471.

- Speakman and Selman, "Physical activity and resting metabolic rate," *Proceedings of the Nutrition Society*, 62 (2003): 621–634.

- Weir, "The exercise effect" *Monitor on Psychology*, 42 (2011): 48.

- Jarolimova, et al., "Obesity: Its epidemiology, comorbidities, and management,"*The Primary Care Companion for CNS Disorders*, 15 (2013): doi: 10.4088/PCC.12f01475.

- Beckman, et al., "Changes in gastrointestinal hormones and leptin after Roux-en-Y gastric bypass procedure: A review," *Journal of the American Dietetic Association*, 110 (2010): 571-584.

- The American Society for Metabolic and Bariatric Surgery provides scientific Information pertaining to bariatric surgery: www.asmbs.org.

- Yanovski and Yanovski, "Long-term drug treatment for obesity: A systematic and clinical review," *Journal of the American Medical Association*, 311 (2014): 74-86.

Chapter 3

- Kwasnicka, et al., "Theoretical explanation for maintenance of behaviour change: A systematic review of behaviour theories." *Health Psychology Review*, 10 (2016): 277-296.

Chapter 4

- Burke, et al., "Self-Monitoring in weight loss: A systematic review of the literature," *Journal of the American Dietetic Association*, 111 (2011): 92-102.

- Helander, et al., "Are breaks in daily self-weighing associated with weight gain?" *PLoS ONE*, 9 (2014): doi:10.1371/journal.pone.0113164.

- Pacanowski, et al., "Daily self-weighing to control body weight in adults: A critical review of the literature," *Sage Open*, 4 (2014): doi:10.1177/2158244014556992.

- Creel, et al., "A randomized trial comparing two interventions to increase physical activity among patients undergoing bariatric surgery," *Obesity*, 24 (2016):1660-1668.

- Archer, et al., "Validity of U.S. nutritional surveillance: National Health and Nutrition Examination Survey caloric energy intake data, 1971-2010," *PLoS ONE*, 8 (2013): doi: 10.1371/journal.pone.0076632

- Cheatham, et al., "The efficacy of wearable activity tracking technology as part of a weight loss program: A systematic review," *The Journal of Sports Medicine and Physical Fitness*, 8 (2017): doi:10.23736/S0022-4707.17.07437-0.

Chapter 5

- Yu, et al., "Metabolic vs. hedonic obesity: A conceptual distinction and its clinical implications," *Obesity*,16 (2015): 234-247.

- Yu, Y-H. "Making sense of metabolic obesity and hedonic obesity," *Journal of Diabetes*, 9 (2017): 656-666.

Chapter 6

- Leehra, et al., "Emotion regulation model in binge eating disorder and obesity--a systematic review," *Neuroscience & Biobehavioral Reviews*, 49 (2015): 125-134.
- Lazarus, et al., "From psychological stress to the emotions: A history of changing outlooks," *Annual Review of Psychology*, 44 (1993): 1-21.
- Cheng, et al., "Improving mental health in health care practioners: Randomized controlled trial of a gratitude intervention," *Journal of Consulting and Clinical Psychology*, 83 (2015):177- 186.
- Koenig, "Research on religion, spirituality, and mental health: A review," *Canadian Journal of Psychiatry*, 54 (2009): 283-291.
- Edenfield and Blumenthal, "Exercise and stress reduction,", in *The Handbook of Stress Science*, ed. Contrada and Baum, Springer Publishing Co., (2011): 301-319.
- Raposa et al., "Prosocial behavior mitigates the negative effects of stress in everyday life," *Clinical Psychological Science*, 4 (2016): 691-698.
- Heijnen et al., "Neuromodulation of aerobic exercise--A review," *Frontiers in Psychology*, (2016): doi:10.3389/fpsyg.2015.01890.

Chapter 7

- Estimated obesity costs to Medicare and Medicaid funding taken from Brookings Institution website, Werman and Harris article entitled "Obesity Costs Evident at the State Level," December 12, 2014. Retrieved August 12, 2017. https://www.brookings.

edu/blog/up-front/2014/12/12/obesity-costs-evident-at-the-state-level/

- Cawley and Maclean, "Unfit for service: The implications of rising obesity for US military recruitment," *Health Economics*, 21 (2012): 1348-1366.

- Wansink, *Mindless Eating*, Bantam Dell, 2006.

Chapters 8-10

- Burns, *The Feeling Good Handbook*, William Morrow and Company, 1989.

- Clark and Beck, *The Anxiety and Worry Workbook*, The Guilford Press, 2012.

- Fairburn, *Overcoming Binge Eating*, The Guilford Press, 2013

- For a summary of types of treatments that work for various psychological disorders see *A Guide to Treatments that Work*. Eds. Nathan and Gorman, Oxford University Press, 2015.

- Lyrics quoted are from "Blue on Black" by the Kenny Wayne Shepherd Band. The song is from the album *Trouble Is…*, released in 1997.

Chapter 11

- Doran, "There's a S.M.A.R.T. Way to Write Management's Goals and Objectives," *Management Review*, 70 (1981): 35-36.

- Wade, "Goal setting in rehabilitation: An overview of what, why and how," *Clinical Rehabilitation*, 23 (2009): 291-295.

- Pearsons, "Goal setting as a health behavior strategy in overweight and obese adults: A systematic literature review examining intervention components," *Patient Education and Counseling*, 87 (2012): 32-42.

Chapter 12

- Kraschnewski,et al., "Long-term weight loss maintenance in the United States," *International Journal of Obesity* 34 (2010): 1644-1654.

- According to baseball-reference.com, 3.7% of official major league at bats were home runs in the 2017 season (retrieved August 13, 2017).

Chapter 13

- Dalrymple, et al., "Diagnosing social anxiety disorder in the presence of obesity: Implications for a proposed change in DSM-5," *Depression and Anxiety*, 28 (2011): 377-382.

- Alberga, et al., Commentary, "Weight bias: A call to action," *Journal of Eating Disorders*, 4 (2016): 1-6.

Index

Acknowledgments

FOR YEARS I enjoyed writing, but never considered myself a writer. Although I'm still not sure about that label, I owe a debt of gratitude to many people who nudged me in that direction. To my small group of writing friends, thanks for reading my work and encouraging me. Enid Cokinos, you were my accountability partner who kept me moving forward with this book. Another special thank you to Julianna Thibodeaux—your style of teaching and editing helped me grow by leaps and bounds. To my editor, Sammie Justesen: I appreciate your patience, wisdom, and guidance. With impeccable timing, you reminded me that our efforts would make someone else's life better.

Many others have helped me by creating time for me to write, encouraging me to persevere, or reassuring me with their interest in this endeavor. You are too many to mention. To my co-workers, friends, colleagues, and family—thank you. I am also especially grateful to the many mentors who helped me throughout the years. Your perspectives taught me about seeking strategies to deal with complex problems and help those around me. I can never repay you for the time you spent with me or the passion you poured into helping me refine my skills.

To my wife, Shana, and my three children—Alden, Mitchell, and Leah--thanks for putting up with me when I was sleep deprived and grumpy or preoccupied with writing, editing, and book cover designs. You fill my life with meaning and purpose.

Lastly, thanks to the many clients I've treated over the years. Your honesty, transparency, and bravery are impressive beyond words. Many of you taught me valuable lessons about resiliency and overcoming obstacles. I'm doing my best to pass these lessons on to others.

About the Author

DR. DAVID CREEL has earned credentials in several disciplines related to weight management. He is a licensed psychologist, an ACSM Certified Clinical Exercise Physiologist, a registered dietitian, and a Certified Diabetes Educator. At Indiana University he completed undergraduate training in dietetics and received bachelor's and master's degrees in exercise science. He received a Ph.D. in clinical psychology from Louisiana State University and trained at the Pennington Biomedical Research Center. Dr. Creel completed his pre-doctoral psychology internship at The Medical University of South Carolina.

Dr. Creel has treated thousands of patients seeking long-term weight loss. Since 2006, he has counseled both bariatric surgery patients and nonsurgical clients at St. Vincent Bariatrics in Carmel, Indiana. His treatment often includes diet and physical activity education, but his main area of focus is helping patients

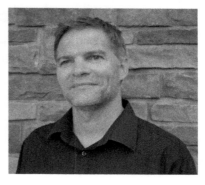

Dr. David Creel

with the psychological aspects of behavior change. He enjoys both individual work and group interventions.

Dr. Creel is also an active researcher. His primary research interests and publications have focused on promoting physical activity among bariatric surgery patients. Dr. Creel enjoys a variety of activities including cycling, competitive table tennis, or a spirited game of cards, or Scrabble. He lives in central Indiana with his wife and their two lovely children.

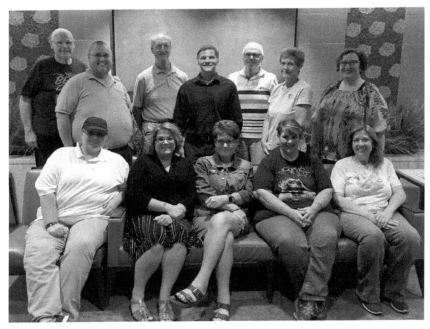

Dr. Creel (second row, center) with a wise group of weight managers

CPSIA information can be obtained
at www.ICGtesting.com
Printed in the USA
LVHW02s1745040118
561822LV00014B/1301/P

9 780997 683462